OXFORD MEDICAL PUBLICATIONS

# Is My Bab

*A Guide for E:*

# Is My Baby All Right?

*A Guide for Expectant Parents*

CHRISTINE GOSDEN
*Department of Obstetrics and Gynaecology,*
*University of Liverpool*

KYPROS NICOLAIDES
*Harris Birthright Research Centre for Fetal Medicine,*
*King's College Hospital, London*

VANESSA WHITTING
*Oxford University Press, Oxford*

OXFORD   NEW YORK   TOKYO
OXFORD UNIVERSITY PRESS
1994

Oxford University Press, Walton Street, Oxford OX2 6DP

Oxford  New York  Toronto
Delhi  Bombay  Calcutta  Madras  Karachi
Kuala Lumpur  Singapore  Hong Kong  Tokyo
Nairobi  Dar es Salaam  Cape Town
Melbourne  Auckland  Madrid
and associated companies in
Berlin  Ibadan

Oxford is a trade mark of Oxford University Press

Published in the United States
by Oxford University Press Inc., New York

A catalogue record for this book is available from the British Library

Library of Congress Cataloging in Publication Data
Gosden, Christine.
Is my baby all right?: a guide for expectant parents/Christine
Gosden, Kypros Nicolaides, Vanessa Whitting.
1. Prenatal diagnosis – Popular works. 2. Prenatal diagnosis –
Moral and ethical aspects. 3. Fetus – Diseases – Popular works
4. Fetus – Abnormalities – Popular works. I. Nicolaides, Kypros.
II. Whitting, Vanessa. III. Title.
RG628.G67 1994    618.3'2-dc20    94-5994
ISBN 0 19 262483 0 (Hbk); ISBN 0 19 262482 2 (Pbk)

Typeset by Advance Typesetting Ltd, Oxfordshire
Printed in Great Britain
by Biddles Ltd
Guildford & King's Lynn

# Preface

'Is my baby all right?' is a question that goes through the mind of every expectant parent – sometimes voiced, sometimes not. Through improvements in medical technology, it is now possible to go a long way towards answering this question before birth. Having such information can be reassuring, or it can present the parents with difficult decisions.

Having said that, the vast majority of pregnancies proceed normally and produce perfectly healthy babies. There are also, inevitably, some babies affected by abnormalities. In a few cases, there is a family history of disease or other risk factor, but in most cases the abnormality seems to happen out of the blue. If you know that you are at risk for a certain condition, you may already know a lot about it and have considered in detail different options relating to testing. Indeed, you may have decided what you want to do if the condition is diagnosed.

You may, however, be one of the many people who have not seen themselves as 'at risk'. An abnormality is picked up through screening tests, and you are then suddenly confronted with a situation where you have to make major decisions about what to do next. Even with the best medical advice, you may feel alone and confused. The arrival of the test results often puts you in the position of making hard choices under pressure of time and without adequate background information. Facts and feelings, medical technology, and strong emotion must be balanced. In these situations, the importance of expert medical counselling and help from family and support groups cannot be overstated. No book can replace these resources. We hope, however, that the information in this book will make the choices more informed, and perhaps easier to live with for being so.

*Liverpool*　　　　　　　　　　　　　　　　　　　　　C.G.
*London*　　　　　　　　　　　　　　　　　　　　　　K.N.
*Oxford*　　　　　　　　　　　　　　　　　　　　　　V.W.
April 1994

# Acknowledgements

First, we would like to thank the parents whose concerns and experiences motivated us to write this book. We would also like to thank our friends and colleagues who provided advice and support throughout the writing period.

Several people deserve special mention for reading numerous drafts. Their input has helped immeasurably with every aspect of the book, and we are very grateful for their time, patience, and expert advice: Professor Chris Higgins, Imperial Cancer Research Fund, Oxford; Dr Ian Young, Dept of Clinical Genetics, City Hospital, Nottingham; Drs Jo Green and Helen Statham, The Cambridge Centre for Family Research, Cambridge; and Dr Theresa Marteau, Wellcome Psychology and Genetics Group, United Medical and Dental Schools of Guy's and St Thomas' Hospitals, London.

# Contents

# Introduction

- *Most babies are born without any noticeable abnormalities.*
- *Prenatal testing is designed to identify abnormalities that do exist as soon and as safely as possible.*
- *You are free to refuse any or all tests.*
- *You may not be offered all the tests that you want.*
- *Testing is not perfect – technology and expertise are improving, but there are limitations.*

This book is about the ways in which abnormalities in babies occur and are detected, and your options relating to diagnosis and afterwards.

The first part of the book (Chapters 1–3) will be useful not only if you are already pregnant, but if you are planning a pregnancy. Chapter 1 introduces the concept of risk, how risks are calculated, and what they mean, as well as the aims of prenatal testing. Chapter 2 provides a brief description of genes and how they work, and the different types of problems that occur when they do not. Chapter 3 explains how environmental factors such as drugs and infections can affect the developing baby.

The second part of the book (Chapters 4 and 5) will be particularly useful if you are already pregnant. Chapter 4 describes the different screening and diagnostic tests and how and why they are performed. Chapter 5 covers the options available if an abnormality is diagnosed.

While you are reading this book, it is worth bearing in mind that most babies are born without any noticeable physical or mental abnormalities. In a book devoted to abnormalities, it can be easy to lose sight of the fact that normal babies make up the majority. On average, only 2–3 per cent of all babies are affected by a serious abnormality. This leaves 97 per cent unaffected. Depending on your outlook, you may either see the half-empty glass instead of the half-full glass, or the doughnut instead of the hole. The aim of this book is to provide you with the framework to make sense of the different influences affecting the way you see your own situation.

If your baby belongs to that 2–3 per cent with a major abnormality, it is of little comfort to know that you are in the minority. If you find yourself in this situation, you will need a clear, concise account of the potential problem and the options available to you. The good news is that a number of such accounts can be provided, thanks to a large amount of scientific and technical progress. It can often be predicted that someone is at higher risk for having an abnormal baby if this has happened before in the family, or if they have been exposed to harmful agents or conditions that are known to cause abnormalities, for example, drugs and infections. Unfortunately, for most people, there are no such predictive factors. This is where prenatal testing comes in – to identify those at higher risk and to detect instances of abnormality before birth.

Prenatal testing should be a service that is offered; it is not mandatory. You are entitled to ask for more information before having any test. You are also free to refuse any or all testing, whether for ethical, religious, or moral reasons, or simply because you are not happy about having the tests. This choice is entirely yours. In theory, you have choices when it comes to the type of test to be performed, but this depends largely on which services are offered in your area. It is not always possible to obtain all the tests you may want because of lack of resources or expertise, or hospital policy.

Some tests carry risks for the baby. Your own perceptions and priorities are what matter. Some parents would see the same test as either reassuring or worrying depending on their own feelings about and experience of abnormality. If you are unhappy with any tests that you are offered, you should discuss your worries with your doctor. The testing procedures, the risks to the baby, and what the results mean are described in Chapter 4.

If you do opt for testing, there are a number of tests that may be performed on everyone (screening tests). These tests are designed to identify in a general way cases where there may be a *potential* problem. Most people with abnormal screening test results will have normal babies, however, and different tests (diagnostic tests) are needed later to distinguish between those babies who are indeed normal and those who have an abnormality.

Many people are uncomfortable with the idea that the doctors caring for them do not have all the answers. Sometimes prenatal testing is an inexact science where much depends on the skill and experience of the people taking and analysing the samples. There is a wide range of abnormalities, some of which are very difficult to describe accurately before birth. The technology is continually improving but there are still many questions, and each new development brings with it new unknowns. For these reasons, it is good to have an understanding of the limitations as well as the benefits of testing and diagnosis.

# 1
# Prenatal testing: questions, answers, and guesses

## MAIN POINTS

- *There are no absolute definitions of 'normal' and 'abnormal'.*
- *Abnormalities that cause disease or disability can have several causes.*
- *Most pregnancies result in a normal baby, but every pregnancy is potentially at risk for abnormality.*
- *Most abnormalities occur in cases where there is no history of the condition in the family.*
- *Your personal risk is determined by your background, genetic make-up, and circumstances. It is reassessed during the pregnancy as test results become known.*
- *Screening tests identify people for whom diagnostic testing is advisable; diagnostic tests give a 'yes' or 'no' answer as to whether the baby is affected by the condition in question.*

## WHAT DOES 'ABNORMAL' MEAN?

Abnormalities range from those that are lethal or cause severe mental or physical disability to those that have few noticeable effects. For the large numbers of conditions in between these two extremes, the word 'serious' is applied differently by different people. It depends on the individual's experience of the condition, perception, and priorities. A doctor who has successfully treated a certain condition might describe it as less 'serious' than a doctor without this experience. If you have a relative with a certain condition, this experience might influence your perception of the situation. Or, if the condition results in a type of disability that you feel you could not live with, you will see it in a different way than someone with different priorities and expectations.

This is one of the hardest things for parents to decide and it is highly personal. If an abnormality is diagnosed, your doctor or genetic counsellor can help in describing what physical or mental effects the condition would have. The questions in the section 'Things you may want to ask' in Chapter 5 are designed to help with your personal decision.

For many conditions, 'normality' and 'abnormality' overlap, and it becomes important to ask, 'what does it mean to be "normal"?' When we see someone walking in the street, we notice whether or not they are within the normal size *range* that we all have in our heads for their age and sex. A similar sort of reckoning goes on in prenatal testing. There are so many factors that vary naturally from parent to parent and baby to baby that it can be very difficult to arrive at precise, absolute definitions of normality. Prenatal tests are designed to establish whether the baby's development is progressing within the wide *range* of what is considered normal. This is done by measuring a variety of factors that are reliable indicators of normal development, which means that the use of 'positive' or 'negative' in reporting test results can be confusing. In testing language, 'negative' is good and means that the baby is not affected by the condition in question, and 'positive' is bad, exactly the opposite of how we usually think. What the result often really means is that the amount or quality of the factor being measured is either inside or outside the normal *range*. For example, the size of the baby's head is often measured on one of the routine ultrasound scans. If the measurement is below the 'average' for the time when the scan is done, there are several explanations aside from the possibility of abnormality. If the estimated date of conception (considered as two weeks after the date of the mother's last menstrual period) is wrong by a week or two, then the baby's head may appear smaller than expected. Even though the measurement fell outside the normal range, the problem lies with the design of the test and not the baby. Even if the dates are right, there are always about 5 per cent of babies with 'abnormally' small head measurements who are not 'abnormal', just small.

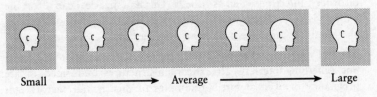

Small ⟶ Average ⟶ Large

Head size range.

'Abnormal' test results do not necessarily mean that there is something wrong with your baby. This depends on many things, including the type of test and whether or not the date of conception has been estimated correctly. Likewise, 'normal' results do not guarantee that there is nothing at all wrong with the baby. Many diseases with a genetic basis are not yet detectable before birth, and some that are detectable are not predictable in their effects. There are also abnormalities without physical signs, and these may not be apparent at birth or even for several years later.

The aim of prenatal testing is not to arrive at definitions of 'normal' and 'abnormal'; the aim is to detect as many serious disorders as safely and as soon as possible. The key thing in all of this is that you should neither despair at abnormal results nor assume that nothing can possibly go wrong if the results of a particular test are normal.

## WHAT ARE THE CAUSES OF ABNORMALITY?

It is not always possible to identify the cause of a particular abnormality. Where it is possible, it is likely to fall into one of the following categories.

1. The baby's chromosomes, the largest unit of genetic material, or a very small part of them (genes – see Chapter 2), are abnormal. This can happen if something went wrong when the parent's sperm or egg was formed or combined, or if the defect has been inherited from one of the parents.

2. The baby's genes and chromosomes are normal but something interferes with the early development of the baby at crucial stages when different parts of the body are being formed. This may either be caused by a lack of essential nutrients or the presence of harmful agents. For example, the lack of certain vitamins is thought to be one of the causes of spina bifida, which results when the nervous system does not develop properly (a 'neural tube defect'). People with spina bifida may have varying degrees of physical disability and learning disorders. Infections such as rubella (German measles) can affect the baby's vision and hearing. Sometimes an excess of a substance such as vitamin A can have a harmful effect as well.

3. The baby's genes, chromosomes, and development may be normal but something interferes after the main structures are formed, in late pregnancy or even at birth. Examples of this include factors that deprive the baby of crucial nutrients or oxygen, such as a placenta

which is not functioning normally. Accidents, prematurity, and labour complications also fall into this category. The abnormality is the result of physical damage or stress to the baby.

Problems can also arise as a result of the complex interactions of genes, personal circumstances, and the environment. One particular abnormality can have several likely causes. For example, spina bifida is linked to a deficiency of the vitamin folic acid and occurs in about 2 pregnancies of every 1000. In some, there may be an explanation, such as,

- *one mother may be malnourished or have an unbalanced diet that is poor in folic acid;*
- *one mother may get plenty of folic acid in her diet but may have a genetic deficiency that prevents her body from absorbing it;*
- *one mother may be taking medication such as anti-epileptic agents that interferes with folic acid absorption;*
- *one mother may be suffering from an illness in which folic acid is not absorbed properly from the digestive tract.*

Likewise, different conditions can arise from the same cause at different stages of development. For example, rubella infection in the first few weeks of pregnancy causes blindness and other complications, but it may cause only deafness if it occurs later on in the fourth month. After this, infection usually does not affect the baby because the critical organs have formed.

## WHO IS AT RISK FOR HAVING A BABY WITH AN ABNORMALITY?

Everyone, absolutely everyone on the planet is at risk. Some of us have a higher risk than others but we are *all* at risk. This is because we all carry faulty genes as evolutionary 'fall-out' (see Chapter 2). We are all vulnerable to hostile factors in the environment and plain bad luck.

Starting with the baseline risk that we all incur as human beings, some people are placed at higher risk by such habits as drinking heavily in pregnancy. Others are routinely exposed to harmful substances such as toxic chemicals or radiation through their jobs. Still others have a higher baseline risk because they belong to an ethnic group with a higher incidence of a particular disease, such as thalassaemia for people of Mediterranean origin or cystic fibrosis for Caucasians. Then there are the people who have a history of genetic disease such as muscular dystrophy in the family. We mention this group last because it is the

**Table 1.1** Known risk groups

---

Mothers who either themselves or a member of their family had a child with

- *a chromosome disorder (for example, Down syndrome)*
- *a genetic disease (for example, cystic fibrosis)*
- *a structural abnormality (for example, cleft palate)*

Older mothers, usually taken as over 35 years old

Mothers who have been exposed to viruses such as rubella (German measles) or HIV or other infections such as toxoplasmosis

Mothers who have been exposed to large amounts of radiation, certain toxic chemicals, or drugs

Mothers with an abnormal early blood test result for a genetic disease (for example, thalassaemia)

Mothers with an abnormal AFP or other blood test result (see Chapter 4)

Mothers with an abnormal ultrasound scan

---

smallest. Contrary to the popular conception that abnormalities result from something 'in the family', more than 90 per cent occur where there is no history of genetic disease. The risk groups that are known to exist are given in Table 1.1.

Screening test results, along with your own particular genetic make-up, habits, background, and circumstances make up your 'individual' risk. The risk you are quoted is an estimate of the chance that an abnormality will arise. As an illustration (see figure p. 9), an average woman with no family history of spina bifida will start off with a base-line risk of 1 in 1000 of having a baby affected by the condition. If she has already had an affected baby, the risk for the current pregnancy increases to 1 in 20; if she has had two affected babies, the risk increases to 1 in 10. If she has a normal blood test result for alpha-fetoprotein (AFP) and a normal ultrasound scan (see Chapter 4), her risk drops nearly to zero.

This example also shows that your risk is constantly revised during the pregnancy. To take another example, a woman who is 37 years old who has had a baby with Down syndrome starts off with a risk of 1 in 100 of it happening again, because the risk of such abnormalities ('chromosomal abnormalities') increases with the mother's age (see figure p. 10 and Table 2.1 p. 24). During pregnancy, test results may

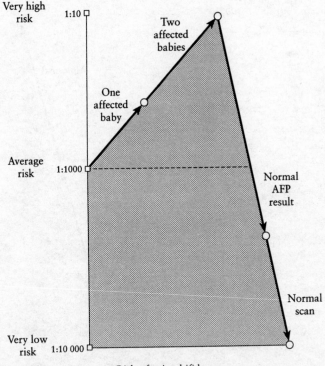

Risk of spina bifida.

cause this risk to be reassessed. Her risk may go down to 1 in 500 after the result of her blood test is known. The ultrasound scan, however, may show certain features associated with chromosomal abnormalities, such as fluid behind the baby's neck, which increases her risk to 1 in 10.

What is 'high' and 'low' in risk terms? Risk, like normality, is a relative concept depending on your starting point. If you start with a very low risk and increase it slightly, you can have a much lower risk than someone with a high baseline risk. The opposite can also be true. For example, a woman with a diet poor in folic acid may still have a lower risk for having a baby with spina bifida than a woman who has a diet rich in folic acid, but who must take medication to control epilepsy.

Risks are quoted as percentages (25 per cent) and as ratios (1:4 or 1 in 4). As well as telling you the chance that your baby will have an abnormality, they also tell you the chance that it will *not*. A risk of 1 in 10, although considered high, still gives a 90 per cent chance that the baby will not be affected by the condition in question. For some

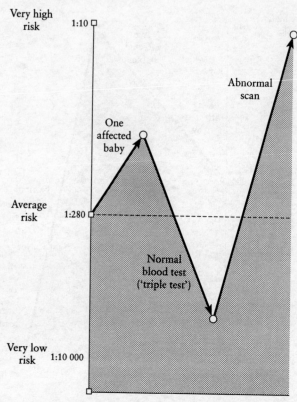

Risk of Down syndrome in a 37-year-old woman.

conditions, the risk that you are quoted will exist for every pregnancy. If, for example, you are quoted an individual risk of 1:4 for cystic fibrosis, and you have already had an affected baby, the same risk still exists for all future pregnancies with the same partner. You cannot 'use up' your bad luck on the first baby or any others. Each time you become pregnant with the same partner you take the same chance. If you change partners, your risk needs to be reassessed.

## WHAT TYPES OF TESTS ARE AVAILABLE?

There are two types of testing method: 'screening' and 'diagnostic'. The different tests in each group are described in Chapter 4. Screening tests are intended to do exactly what the name implies, to identify mothers

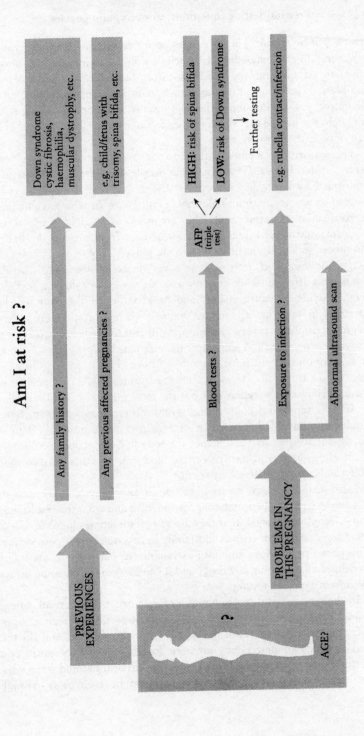

# Am I at risk ?

Down syndrome
cystic fibrosis,
haemophilia,
muscular dystrophy, etc.

e.g. child/fetus with
trisomy; spina bifida, etc.

Any family history ?

Any previous affected pregnancies ?

PREVIOUS
EXPERIENCES

AGE?

?

HIGH: risk of spina bifida

LOW: risk of Down syndrome

Further testing

e.g. rubella contact/infection

AFP
(triple
test)

Blood tests ?

Exposure to infection ?

Abnormal ultrasound scan

PROBLEMS IN
THIS PREGNANCY

who *might* be at risk. They are often performed routinely for everyone attending the antenatal clinic and include simple and inexpensive things such as establishing the family medical history and taking blood samples. A common misconception is that screening tests lead to a definitive 'yes' or 'no' about the condition in question. Screening tests highlight the people for whom further testing is advisable – those who fall outside the 'normal' range.

The majority of women with abnormal screening results have perfectly normal babies. However, some people will have an abnormality confirmed by later, diagnostic tests. Diagnostic tests are usually only offered to women with an identifiable risk factor or who have had an abnormal screening test result. They are more complicated and costly to perform, and involve taking samples of cells from around the baby. Amniocentesis and chorionic villus sampling (CVS) are examples of diagnostic tests. Such tests provide a 'yes' or 'no' answer as to whether the baby is affected by the condition in question. They do not, on their own, provide a picture of how and to what degree the baby will be affected. In some cases, such as Down syndrome or spina bifida, the degree of disability is very variable and difficult to predict. Doctors must use their experience and judgement to determine the 'prognosis' – what the condition will mean for the baby's future. This is one reason why, even if you are totally at ease with the idea of testing, it is important to have a balanced awareness of what the tests can and cannot tell you.

Another important point is that several different tests are sometimes needed to confirm the existence of a suspected abnormality. This is partly due to the fact that neither the tests nor the people performing them are perfect, and partly because there can be other reasons than abnormality for 'positive' test results.

Most people are now aware of testing in some way, and are anxious to varying degrees about what the tests involve and what the results may show. People who know that they are at risk sometimes hide the fact of their pregnancy from friends and family in case something goes wrong. This puts a tremendous amount of strain on the parents who are trying to behave as if nothing is wrong, and it can be resolved to some degree by certain types of testing.

In the simplest and most common case, a negative test result brings immediate and welcome reassurance. **It is important to realize, however, that a 'negative' result means only that the problem that the test was designed to detect has not been found.** It does not mean that nothing else can happen. This is a hard thing to bear in mind when what you desperately want is reassurance; it can be even more painful,

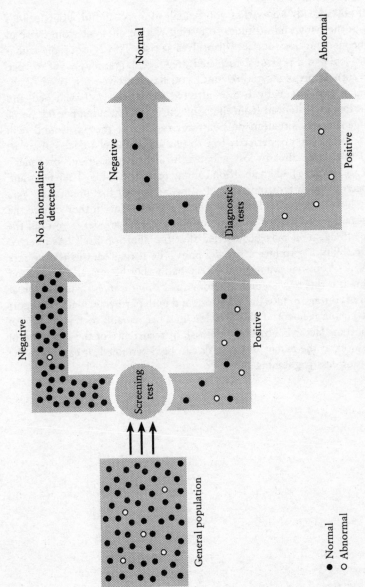

Screening and diagnosis.

General population

Screening test

Negative

No abnormalities detected

Positive

Diagnostic tests

Negative

Normal

Positive

Abnormal

- Normal
- Abnormal

however, to be shocked later on if you have convinced yourself that nothing can go wrong.

If you already know that you belong to a risk group, your feelings about the baby and attitudes to testing will be different from those of someone who does not see themselves at risk. This is especially true if you have had a previously affected pregnancy. You may want to keep the current pregnancy secret until you have received test results confirming that the baby is not affected. You may feel detached and emotionally distanced from the baby during this waiting period. Some women in this situation do not want to look at the ultrasound scan image, and you are perfectly free to refuse if you feel anxious about it.

If you have already lost a baby through a miscarriage or genetic disease, or have had an abortion for any reason, you may have fears and concerns that differ from those of someone in their first pregnancy. You may have been through the tests before and wonder if they caused the miscarriage, or elected to have an abortion and wonder if you did the right thing. You may be worried that the abortion itself has affected your ability to produce a healthy baby. (Be reassured: this is very rare indeed.) You may want a baby very badly, but be apprehensive about losing it if this has happened before one or more times. It takes a great deal of courage to face the situation, and both partners will need support and encouragement if the decision has been made to try again. An important factor is obviously the risk of recurrence of the condition in question. If the extent of this risk can be determined, it can make the decision less frightening.

# 2
# Genes: how they work and what happens when they don't

## MAIN POINTS

- *Genes control the function of all systems in the body.*
- *We all carry abnormal genes, most of which are not noticeable, because of evolutionary change.*
- *Abnormalities that cause disease or disability can result from several types of genetic error.*
- *The type of disorder determines the choice of prenatal tests and the recurrence risk.*
- *For some conditions, the same risk applies to any future pregnancy with the same partner.*

## HOW THEY WORK

Genes carry the instructions that determine every single trait and control the functioning of every system in the body, from the colour of your hair to the production of the substances in your stomach that help you to digest food. Some genes work alone, others in combination; some control the development of the baby, some its skin colour. Every physical trait is controlled, either completely or partly, by the combination of the mother's and father's genes. Certain environmental factors can also affect the way that genes work and these are described in Chapter 3.

The smallest unit of a gene is the 'base'. Bases combine in pairs and each pair is joined to the next in an infinitely variable sequence, forming the long double helix that is known as DNA (deoxyribonucleic acid). The order of the bases provides the code that the cells of your body follow to produce the different proteins that they need.

Genes are the functional units of DNA, and each one provides the code for a different protein. Genes may be thousands of bases long, and they are arranged in a specific pattern, linked together, and coiled tightly to form chromosomes. Every cell in the body (except sperm and egg cells – see below) has thousands of genes organized on to 46 chromosomes, which in turn are arranged in 23 pairs. Thus, there are two copies of each gene, one on each member of each pair (see diagram). This is very important to remember because all of the baby's traits and characteristics are determined by the interaction of the copies of the genes received from the mother and father.

These terms – base, gene, chromosome – simply refer to different levels of packaging of the DNA, the 'genetic material' of the cell. There are several useful metaphors for the distinctive double helix structure (a zipper, a staircase, a ladder) and the function (building blocks, a blueprint, a secret code) of DNA. Regardless of which image works best for you, the important thing to bear in mind is that DNA controls the development of your baby and therefore anything that interferes with it poses a potential risk.

Many people have been told that the DNA in our cells usually produces an exact duplicate when it divides, so what is responsible for the amazing diversity that exists in nature? Why don't we all look the same if we have exact copies of our parent's genes? It is true that all of the cells in the body **except for eggs and sperm** usually make exact copies of themselves when they divide. Eggs and sperm are produced through a different process where the genetic material is split between two cells, giving each of them just 23 chromosomes. The chromosomes physically exchange pieces of themselves with their opposite number during this process, reshuffling and rearranging to result in a totally new combination each time. Sperm meets egg and, if all goes well, fuse to make a new, unique set of 46 chromosomes, one member of each pair from the mother and one from the father. Anything other than 46, or any genetic sequence that is not 100 per cent normal, has the potential to cause problems. It is during this reshuffling that chromosomes can sometimes be damaged, or the numbers of chromosomes altered, leading to a variety of problems for the baby. The diagram opposite (see figure p. 17) below illustrates these processes, known as mitosis and meiosis.

This genetic reshuffling works as a powerful evolutionary force by introducing new traits that may be useful in helping species to cope with pressures in the environment. If a new trait or 'mutation' that has a beneficial effect is generated by this reshuffling, it will be 'selected'. This means that it will become a permanent resident in the DNA unless or until something better comes along. Take the giraffe as an example. The first one who had, by chance, a slightly longer neck than the others would be better able to eat the leaves out of their reach, which could

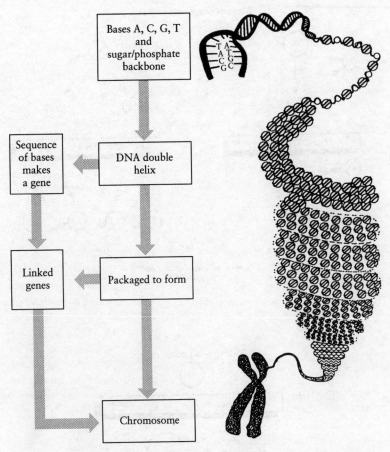

Chromosomes, genes, and DNA.

have conferred on it several advantages – stronger and better able to outrun a predator, more likely to survive the next drought – all of which would enhance its chances of reproducing successfully. According to evolutionary theory, this would result in the genes for longer necks being 'selected'.

How is this talk of genes and giraffes relevant to prenatal testing? Taking all of the above into account, it should not be surprising that more than 90 per cent of genetic disorders arise out of the blue in people who are not linked to any risk factor. The common perception is just the opposite – that most cases occur when there is something 'in the family'. The fact is that the majority of disorders happen as totally

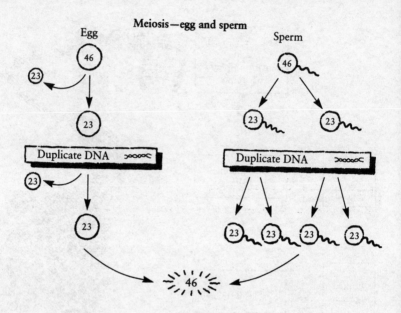

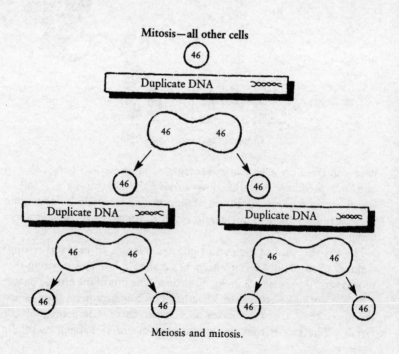

Meiosis and mitosis.

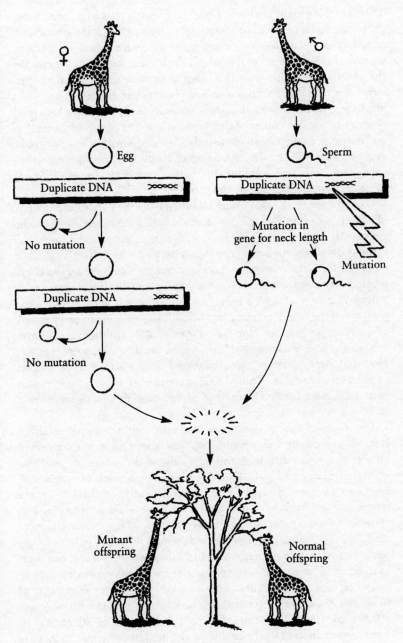

Mutation of neck-length gene.

unpredictable genetic mistakes. Different prenatal tests work at different packaging levels of the genetic material to try and detect these mistakes, including using ultrasound scanning to get extra visual evidence of structural abnormalities in the baby. In chromosome tests, for example, the chromosomes are stained so that their numbers, overall shapes, structures, and characteristic banding patterns can be seen. These tests are done to detect abnormalities that result from problems at a high level – extra or missing copies of chromosomes, pieces of chromosome that are missing, damaged, stuck together, or appearing the wrong way around. They will not detect missing or faulty individual genes, which can only be found by using other tests that look at the level of the gene or at the protein encoded by the gene.

For most genes, the two copies inherited from the parents are similar. However, as a result of the evolutionary forces described above, some genes exist in more than one form, a 'dominant' form and a 'recessive' form. A dominant copy of a gene shows itself or is 'expressed' regardless of which form the other copy takes. A recessive copy of a gene is expressed only when it is paired with another recessive. If it is paired with a dominant copy of a gene it may be invisible, or it may affect the expression of the dominant copy (see below). It is possible to carry a copy of the recessive gene for blue eyes, for example, even though your eyes are brown. If your partner has brown eyes, but also carries the recessive blue-eyed form, you may have a blue-eyed child if it receives two copies of the blue-eyed form. Thus different traits have different inheritance patterns that are labelled 'dominant' or 'recessive' depending on the type of gene involved.

The forces of change that result in neutral mutations such as differences in eye colour and advantageous mutations such as long-necked giraffes can also result in harmful mutations that cause physical disability, disease, or mental impairment. We do not think of people with blue eyes as being affected by a 'recessive genetic condition', yet the inheritance mechanism for blue eyes is the same as for a disease such as cystic fibrosis (CF). Parents who carry one copy of the recessive form of the CF gene are not affected by the condition. If they each pass on a copy of the recessive form of the gene to the baby, however, it will definitely be affected. There are also some cases where it can be an advantage to carry one copy of a defective recessive gene. This is true in the case of sickle cell disease and beta thalassaemia, where people with only one affected copy of the gene are described as 'carriers' of the condition. They are not affected by the condition and are more resistant to malaria than people with two normal copies of the gene. This random change,

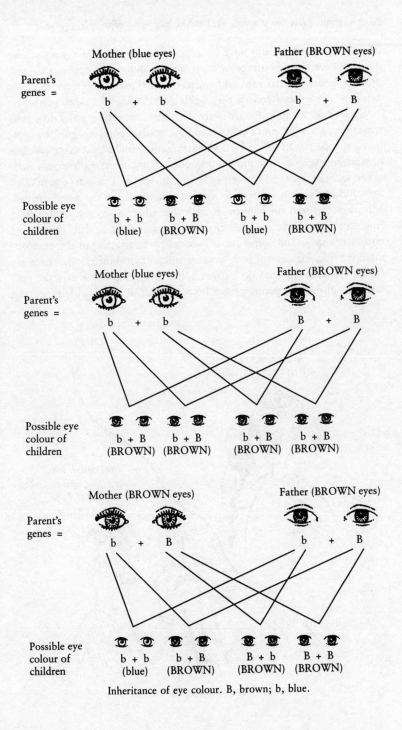

Inheritance of eye colour. B, brown; b, blue.

when it occurred, would have been beneficial in tropical areas such as Africa where the advantage of carrying one defective copy of the gene (greater resistance to malaria) outweighed the risk of receiving two defective copies and contracting sickle cell disease or thalassaemia.

We are not normally aware of the different things that genes do unless something goes wrong. The total human genetic complement (the 'genome') comprises 33 000 000 000 bases, which includes a large amount of material whose function is unknown. Some sections are repeated, other sections seem to be simply filling up space. The active genes, all 200 000 of them, are normally copied exactly each time a cell divides. Mistakes can and do happen at all levels when genes are copied – a single base, a single gene, a miscopied sequence, a broken or missing chromosome – and some are influenced by substances in the environment outside our control such as radiation and viral infection. There are repair mechanisms that do correct some mistakes. If the mistake prevents an important protein from being produced in a usable form, the

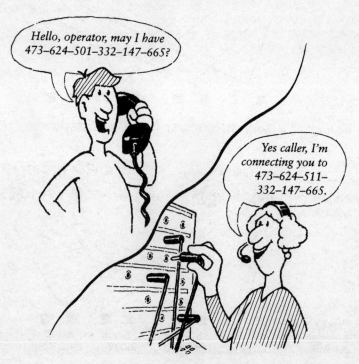

If genes were like telephone numbers.

consequences of even a single incorrect base can lead to serious problems. This is the case for sickle cell disease. In this disease, the molecule that transports oxygen in the bloodstream (haemoglobin) is affected as the result of a single base change that alters the site on the molecule where oxygen attaches. It is astonishing to think that the change of a single base among the millions of bases in the DNA could cause such a debilitating disease. What is even more amazing is that mistakes do not occur more often. Imagine if telephone numbers had millions of digits and had to be copied exactly each time you wanted to make a call. Most of us would never talk to anyone, yet overall the frequency of genetic errors that result in serious disease is relatively low.

Parents often feel that they must be to blame somehow, that they are unique in having 'faulty' genes. The problem actually affects a huge proportion of the population in an incredibly wide variety of ways. This does not mean that everyone without a known genetic disorder has faultless genes; everyone has 'faulty genes' in one way or another, but most of us live our lives happily unaware of this. We are all carrying around numerous genetic errors without there being any noticeable effect. Such people appear 'normal' in every way, and one is probably sitting next to you right now. The difference between these individuals and those affected by genetic disease is nothing more than luck. Thus, the idea of discriminating against genetically 'abnormal' people rapidly becomes absurd.

## THE THINGS THAT GO WRONG

This section deals with the instances where genetic errors do result in disease. There may be too few or too many chromosomes; the chromosomes may have been damaged or rearranged in a harmful way when the egg or sperm was formed; a new mutation may have arisen when the DNA was copied; or a harmful mutation may have been inherited from one of the parents.

### Chromosome disorders

Normally, we have 23 pairs of chromosomes, making a total of 46. Chromosome disorders are characterized by a change in either the total number of chromosomes or in the amount of genetic material they contain, less or more. Down syndrome is the best known chromosome disorder, but there are many others, which vary in their effects. Some types are lethal and result in miscarriage, often before the woman knows

**Table 2.1** Maternal age-specific rates for chromosome abnormalities*

| Maternal age (years) | Risk of | |
|---|---|---|
| | Down syndrome | All chromosome abnormalities |
| 35 | 1 in 286 | 1 in 78 |
| 36 | 1 in 175 | 1 in 71 |
| 37 | 1 in 147 | 1 in 66 |
| 38 | 1 in 123 | 1 in 60 |
| 39 | 1 in 92 | 1 in 48 |
| 40 | 1 in 81 | 1 in 42 |
| 41 | 1 in 68 | 1 in 35 |
| 42 | 1 in 45 | 1 in 22 |
| 43 | 1 in 31 | 1 in 20 |
| 44 | 1 in 33 | 1 in 22 |
| 45 | 1 in 22 | 1 in 14 |
| 46 | 1 in 12 | 1 in 10 |

* Based on amniocentesis data.

she is pregnant. Other lethal chromosome disorders are responsible for later miscarriage, stillbirth, or death during the first few days or months after birth. Some serious chromosome disorders are not lethal, but cause major physical and mental disability. At the other end of the spectrum, there are many chromosome disorders that have comparatively few, if any, noticeable effects.

Little is known about the factors that cause chromosome disorders, apart from the increased risk for older mothers (see Table 2.1). In the vast majority of cases, the chromosomes of the parents are normal, but something goes wrong when the egg or sperm is being formed. In a few cases the problem actually exists in the chromosomes of one of the parents. In this instance, the affected parent looks perfectly normal because the total amount of genetic material that they are carrying is normal. Because it is arranged in the wrong way, however, it can be passed on in an unbalanced form.

TRISOMIES

More is not better when dealing with chromosomes; the normal condition is 'disomy' – a pair of each, one from the mother and one from the father. An extra or 'trisomy' of chromosome number 21, for example, causes Down syndrome. Aside from the mental retardation associated with Down syndrome, affected children sometimes have other problems including heart defects. Before the use of antibiotic treatment and heart surgery, many children with this condition used to die in infancy from chest infections and heart problems. Some babies die in childhood and some people may live to be 60, but the average age of survival is now 20 years. In Edward syndrome there is an extra copy of chromosome 18. Many babies with this condition are stillborn, but some can survive several weeks or even months. The babies suffer from growth retardation, brain defects, cleft lip and palate, heart defects, kidney and bladder problems, and deformed hands and feet. Patau syndrome, which is due to an extra copy of chromosome 13, is similar to Edward syndrome in terms of poor survival and the presence of several abnormalities.

## TRIPLOIDY

It is even possible to receive three copies of not one, but *every* chromosome, making a total of 69 instead of 46; this is known as 'triploidy'. Some cases arise by accident when an egg is fertilized by two sperms, but some errors occur when the egg or sperm is formed. Triploid babies are usually stillborn or die within a couple of days after birth.

## SEX CHROMOSOME ABNORMALITIES

There are several disorders affecting the chromosomes that determine the sex of the baby, the X and Y chromosomes, and, taken together, they are relatively common. Females normally have XX and males have XY, but it is possible to end up with an extra sex chromosome. Most people with sex chromosome abnormalities have IQs in the normal range and develop normally. The effects include:

- 47 XXX (triple X females who may have behavioural and educational problems);
- 47 XXY (Klinefelter syndrome where males are usually infertile);
- 47 XYY (males who have an extra Y and may have behavioural problems).

Another sex chromosome disorder is Turner syndrome (45 X) where females have only one rather than two X chromosomes. About 90 per cent of affected babies die before birth; those who survive are infertile, tend to be short and may have heart abnormalities.

TRANSLOCATIONS/REARRANGEMENTS

There are a number of conditions that result when chromosomes, or parts of chromosomes, swap positions or otherwise rearrange themselves when the egg and sperm are forming. It is possible for one of the parents to have a 'balanced' form of such an abnormality that does not cause any problems when it is passed on to the baby in the same form. If such a balanced chromosome abnormality is mixed up when the egg or sperm is formed, however, it is possible that the baby will receive too much or too little genetic material. The extent of the physical and mental disability that might affect the baby depends on the exact arrangement of the chromosomes and whether material has been lost or gained.

## Single gene disorders

Single gene disorders are caused by one or more abnormal genes being passed on from parent to child, or by a new mutation which arises when the egg or sperm is formed.

There are three main categories of disorders where the condition is caused by a single defective gene: dominant, X-linked or sex-linked, and recessive.

DOMINANT

Only one copy of the defective gene from either parent is needed to cause disease. Only one parent may show symptoms of the disease but sometimes these defective genes may arise as new mutations and the parent is unaffected. There is a 1 in 2 chance of passing on the disease to either male or female children. For severe conditions where people are infertile or do not survive long enough to have children, all cases arise as new mutations.

In large families it is sometimes possible to trace a disease from an affected parent to about half of all their children (boys and girls), and such pedigrees show clear evidence of the dominant inheritance of a single gene disorder. Only one copy of a defective dominant gene is needed to cause the disease because it overwhelms the normal, recessive copy. In such cases, it is possible to see that an affected person has a 1 in 2 chance of passing on the disease to their child.

Examples of dominantly inherited diseases include achondroplasia (dwarfism) and Huntington's chorea, the inheritance pattern for which is illustrated opposite (see figure p. 27).

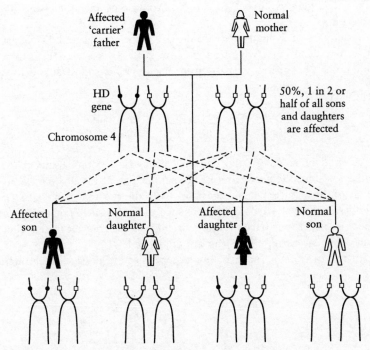

Inheritance of Huntington's chorea (HC).

## X-LINKED OR SEX-LINKED RECESSIVE

These conditions are inherited from a carrier mother (or may arise as new mutations), who usually shows few or no symptoms herself, by 50 per cent of male babies. Half of her daughters will be carriers themselves and have few or no symptoms. Males who are affected by an X-linked disease will not have affected sons because the sons receive the father's Y chromosome. All the daughters of affected males will be carriers because they receive the father's affected X chromosome.

Bearing in mind that the sex chromosomes that characterize females are XX and XY for males, it is understandable how a defective gene on a female's X chromosome can be hidden. If her other X chromosome is normal, the carrier mother will not show the effects of the defective copy because they are masked by the normal one. Males, however, have only one X chromosome, so the disease trait is expressed if they inherit the defective X from their mother. Thus, the picture becomes clearer if, for example, a brother has the disease and his three sisters all have affected sons. The gene is 'linked' to the X chromosome that their sons are inheriting.

Examples of X-linked conditions are haemophilia and Duchenne muscular dystrophy, where about 1 in 3 cases is caused by a new mutation. The inheritance pattern for haemophilia is illustrated below.

## RECESSIVE

Two copies of the defective gene, one from each parent, are needed to cause disease. Parents do not usually show signs of the disease themselves.

A child must inherit the defective gene from both parents to be affected. Since the gene is recessive, neither parent usually shows any signs of the disease, but together they carry the risk that 1 in 4 of their children will be affected. A '1 in 4 chance' exists for *every* pregnancy for that couple; if they have an affected child, it does not mean that they can count on having three who are unaffected.

In this way, a harmful recessive gene may be passed on through

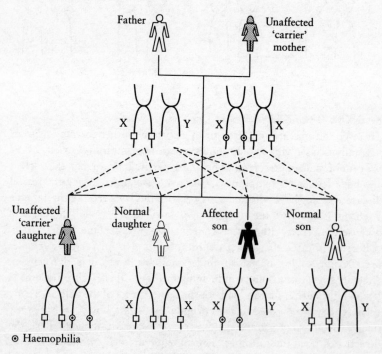

Inheritance of haemophilia.

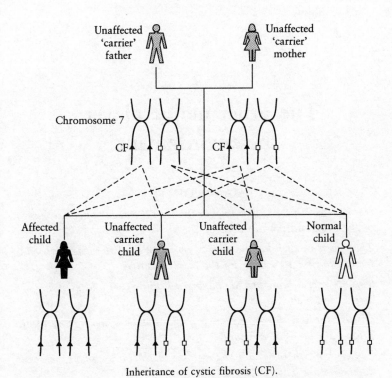

Inheritance of cystic fibrosis (CF).

several generations without anyone having the symptoms of the condition. New recessive mutations may take a long time to show in a population because the disease only arises when two carriers have an affected child. In such cases, there is a much greater chance that people who are closely related will both carry the same abnormal gene. This is the basis for our taboo against marriage between cousins, as this increases the chance that two copies of the same abnormal recessive gene will be passed on to their children. The risk exists in any community where a particular gene occurs very frequently. The occurrence of some recessive conditions varies between ethnic groups. In Caucasian populations, about 1 person in 20 is a carrier of the recessive gene for cystic fibrosis (inheritance pattern given above), and in Mediterranean populations, as many as 1 in 10 people may carry the recessive gene for beta thalassaemia without actually showing any symptoms of the disease themselves. For these conditions there are many mutations, and carriers of two different mutations in the same gene may actually have an affected child.

# 3
# The other major player: the environment

## MAIN POINTS

- *Some factors in the environment can affect the developing baby; most of these are outside our control.*
- *The effects of such factors depend on when the baby was exposed to them; the first 10 weeks are the most sensitive.*
- *Sensible precautions include having a healthy diet and avoiding cigarettes and alcohol.*
- *Discuss the use of medication for illness with your doctor, ideally before you become pregnant.*
- *If you think there is any chance you might be pregnant, tell your doctor before having X-rays for anything.*
- *Most women have been immunized against the common infections by the time they become pregnant.*
- *There are routine screening tests for some infections; other tests may be recommended if infection occurs for the first time during pregnancy.*
- *Multifactorial conditions result from the combination of genetic and environmental factors.*

Now that we have been through the ways in which faulty genes can be inherited, it is time to look at the other major influence on the baby's development: the environment. You have some choices regarding such things as diet, smoking, and drinking, but even healthy, so-called 'clean-living' people can have abnormal babies. It may happen as a result of a random mutation, or as a consequence of exposure to drugs, radiation, or infection. It may also be due to a combination of a mutation and something from outside. However, it is important to note that influences in the environment account for only around 10 per cent of all developmental defects. We have included a fair amount of detail because, unlike genetic abnormalities, some can potentially be avoided and you should be aware of possible testing methods for others.

The effects of environmental factors on the baby are related to the developmental stage at which the exposure occurred. The most sensitive stretch of time is during the first 10 weeks of gestation because most of the major organs form during this time and spend the rest of the pregnancy growing and beginning to function. The timing for each step is critical, and the whole complicated sequence can be disrupted by changes in timing or missed steps. Imagine a very highly sophisticated factory, such as one in which cars are manufactured. If something disrupts the production process, it can have a large or small effect, depending upon what part of the car is being built when the disruption occurs. If something distorts the chassis while it is being formed, it may be difficult or impossible to assemble the rest of the car. If a piece of interior trim is missing or broken, however, the effects are less serious.

While the baby is developing, there are four types of circumstances that can cause abnormalities: teratogens, infections, combinations of different factors, and pregnancy complications and accidents in labour.

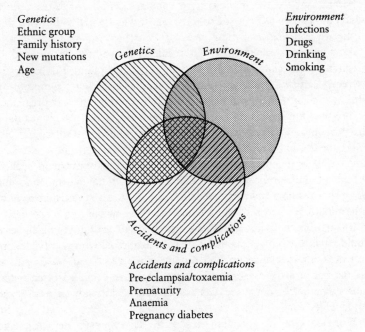

*Genetics*
Ethnic group
Family history
New mutations
Age

*Environment*
Infections
Drugs
Drinking
Smoking

*Accidents and complications*
Pre-eclampsia/toxaemia
Prematurity
Anaemia
Pregnancy diabetes

Relationship between genetics, the environment, and accidents and complications.

## TERATOGENS

Normal development can be disrupted if the baby is exposed to a harmful agent such as a virus, a drug, radiation, an excess of a naturally occurring substance such as a vitamin, or chemicals (including alcohol). Agents that have such effects are known as 'teratogens'. They come from outside and interfere with the baby's development; there may well be nothing wrong with either the baby's or the parents' genes or chromosomes. The important thing to remember is that the effect of a particular teratogen will depend on when it appears during the developmental process.

## *Drugs and medicines*

The story of thalidomide has had a dramatic effect on the general awareness of the risks from drugs and medicines in pregnancy. In the early 1960s thalidomide was widely prescribed to alleviate morning sickness. A large number of women had taken the drug before reports of abnormalities began to appear. In some cases, only the tips of fingers or toes were missing, but some doctors reported cases of missing limbs. It became apparent that the type of damage was related to the time at which the baby was exposed to the drug. It was finally withdrawn first in the US and then in Britain.

As a general rule, drugs and medications should be avoided in pregnancy, especially in the first 3 months, but taking this policy to extremes can also be dangerous. Many women experience symptoms of illness, such as urinary tract infections and vomiting, in early pregnancy before they know that they are pregnant. It rarely happens that taking drugs such as anti-emetics, most antibiotics, and pain killers has any effect on the baby. However, severe vomiting can, if untreated, have adverse effects itself on the baby because of the loss of nutrients such as folic acid. Furthermore, extreme anxiety about having an abnormal baby as a result of taking medication can lead to the decision to have a termination, even if nothing is proven to be wrong.

If you think that you have been exposed to a drug or anything else that could harm the baby, it is best to tell your doctor, who will be able to consult with specialists to find out what the risks really are. This is crucial because the stage at which the exposure occurred often determines whether or not there was any damage at all, as well as the type of damage.

Women with chronic illnesses such as epilepsy, diabetes, and Crohn's disease often have to take medication regularly, and it would be dangerous to discontinue this. If you are planning a pregnancy and are taking medication, ideally you should consult your doctor before you conceive. Drug regimes can be modified in pregnancy to achieve the best balance of managing the mother's disease with minimum risk to the baby. Some drugs can cross the placenta while others cannot. For example, thrombosis is a condition that is treated with drugs that help to prevent blood clots. The drug warfarin can be taken in tablet form, which is convenient, but it can cross the placenta and cause abnormalities if taken in the first trimester of pregnancy. If taken later in pregnancy, it can cause brain haemorrhage in the baby. Heparin must be given as one or two injections per day, which is uncomfortable and inconvenient, but it does not cross the placenta. Thus, if you suffer from thrombosis during pregnancy, only heparin is safe to take.

ILLICIT DRUGS

Cocaine has been shown to have serious effects on the developing nervous system and heart, amounting to an almost 10-fold increase in the risk of abnormality over women who do not use the drug. It is also associated with a higher risk of prematurity, stillbirth, and spontaneous abortion. Facial abnormalities and behavioural problems are seen in surviving infants. The effects are most significant if the baby is exposed to the drug in the first 3 months. Other drugs such as heroin, crack, ecstasy, etc. are also highly dangerous to the baby. There appears to be no connection between smoking marijuana and abnormalities.

CONTRACEPTIVES

Many women discover that they are pregnant while they are still using contraceptives and become concerned that the contraceptives – the Pill, spermicides, the coil (IUD) – could affect their baby. The risk from taking the Pill in the first trimester is considered to be very small indeed, but there have been conflicting studies on the subject. If your period is late, you should have a pregnancy test before starting your next pack of pills. Vaginal spermicides do not pose any increased risk of abnormality, nor does the coil. If you become pregnant with a coil in place, you run a higher risk of miscarriage, but not of abnormality.

Some drugs such as progesterone are prescribed for women who have had miscarriages in the past or if there is bleeding in the current pregnancy. Some progesterones resemble the male hormone testosterone, it can have a masculinizing effect on a female baby's genitalia.

## Cigarette smoking

Even if you are not taking any kind of medication or drug, you could be exposing your baby to harmful substances through your habits. Smokers are twice as likely to have a spontaneous abortion as non-smokers, and have more premature and low-birth-weight babies. This risk increases with the number of cigarettes smoked. One study has also shown that passive smoking can increase the risk of having a low-birth-weight baby. Sudden infant death syndrome (cot death) is also associated with smoking, but it is not clear if this is due to smoking during pregnancy or after. If you and/or your partner are able to stop smoking before and during pregnancy, the effects of all of these factors are reduced.

## Alcohol

Alcohol can have major effects on the development of your baby. It can cause growth retardation both before and after birth, facial abnormalities, some mental retardation, and learning disorders. The effects increase with the amount of alcohol consumed. However, there are no clear correlations between the amount drunk and the type of damage that results. This is because the effects are related to the mother's metabolism, her weight and age, and particularly her ability to remove the toxic by-products of alcohol breakdown. These can have severe effects on the developing brain and other organs if consumed at critical periods such as the third and tenth weeks. At other times, steady drinking can lower the birthweight and/or the IQ of the baby. It is good to remember that if you feel tipsy, your baby may be drunk.

Many women find alcohol unpalatable during pregnancy. If you do not, even if you are a heavy drinker you will lessen the damage to the baby by cutting down as soon as possible.

## X-rays

The use of X-rays has had a major impact on modern medicine, yet radiation was still poorly understood when X-rays first came into use for the diagnosis and treatment of disease. The doses of X-rays that we now receive for routine procedures are several times lower than in the 1920s and 1930s, when large doses were used to treat pelvic disease. Precautions, such as covering the rest of the body with a lead apron, are also taken to expose only the part of the body where the problem is suspected. So, if you need an X-ray for a broken leg, nothing else but your leg is exposed. It is entirely safe to have your teeth X-rayed; indeed, you are advised to see your dentist regularly while you are pregnant anyway because of the demands that your baby makes on your calcium supplies. It is also safe to go through airport security archways.

If you do need an X-ray of the abdomen the risk of damage is low, but you should *always* tell your doctor and the radiographer if you think you are pregnant. It is thought that children whose mothers had abdominal X-rays while they were pregnant stand a 1 in 2000, instead of 1 in 3000, chance of developing leukaemia later in life. However, it would be a tragedy if women were advised to have terminations on this basis because 2000 pregnancies would be terminated to 'prevent' a single case of leukaemia.

# INFECTIONS

We have covered infections in detail for your information because many people have heard of cases of abnormality resulting from infections, but this is actually a relatively uncommon occurrence. Many women are immune to viruses such as rubella and cytomegalovirus (CMV) by the time they become pregnant. Very few women are both susceptible and exposed to the rarer viruses.

## CHICKENPOX/SHINGLES

These diseases are both caused by the varicella-zoster virus. Abnormalities are very uncommon, but when they do occur they can be serious. These include missing limbs, paralysis, and mental retardation. If infection occurs within 5 days of delivery, it can be passed on to the baby, and the results of this are sometimes fatal. If you show the symptoms of chickenpox infection, a detailed ultrasound scan will be done to look for structural effects. Later on, a fetal blood sample (see Chapter 4) can be done to confirm infection in the baby. There is also a vaccine that can reduce the effects of the disease for you and the baby.

Infection with herpes zoster (shingles), on the other hand, has not been shown to result in abnormalities.

## CYTOMEGALOVIRUS (CMV)

This is a common virus that usually produces no symptoms or, at most, symptoms like those of a mild attack of influenza. It can be transmitted to the baby through the placenta and through breast milk. Most women will have had the virus before they become pregnant and have antibodies that can cross the placenta and partially protect the baby if re-infection occurs during pregnancy. If, however, infection occurs for the first time during pregnancy, no antibodies will be present and in approximately 10 per cent of cases the virus crosses the placenta, resulting in serious problems. There is no specific screening test for CMV infection. If certain abnormalities are detected on the ultrasound scan, a series of tests can be done to determine if infection has been passed to the baby. The good news is that new technology is being developed that should aid in the definite diagnosis of this virus, and also few women reach their child-bearing years without already having had the virus. The only advice offered is to practice strict personal hygiene. This may sound obvious, but it is especially important if you come into contact with children or infants regularly because they can have active infections.

## HERPES SIMPLEX VIRUS (HSV)

Many people suffer from genital herpes infection, but the place of the disease in the media has been taken over completely by HIV and AIDS. The disease is sexually transmitted and is characterized by painful genital ulcers. The symptoms come and go but the infection is permanent. For pregnant women who are infected, it is very rare for the disease to be transmitted to the baby in the womb. Infection can, however, be passed on as a result of contact with active lesions on the mother's genitals during delivery. (A Caesarean section would be recommended in these cases but, if no ulcers can be seen, then vaginal delivery would be safe.) As the consequences of infection by this route can be serious and even fatal, babies who survive may have abnormalities of the nervous system. Thus it is very important to tell the medical staff if you have herpes. Infection in the mother can be diagnosed from samples taken of the ulcers. HSV cannot be transmitted through breast milk.

## HIV (HUMAN IMMUNODEFICIENCY VIRUS)

HIV is the virus associated with AIDS and infection ultimately weakens the immune system to the point where other infections can invade. People do not 'die of AIDS'; they die of diseases that invade after the virus has damaged their immune defences. There is a long 'latent' period, often lasting several years, in which there are no symptoms.

The virus cannot penetrate unbroken skin – it needs direct access to the bloodstream through breaches in the skin surface. This is known to happen primarily amongst those who inject drugs or practice anal sex, and women who have high numbers of sexual partners may be at greater risk. Infection is becoming more common, however, among people who do not belong to any of these groups. Antibodies are produced in response to infection by HIV, but these do not affect the virus. As yet there exists neither a cure nor a vaccine.

There is a risk of about 30 per cent of transmitting the disease to the baby. If the baby is infected, the illness may not develop until around 8 months of life, and the average survival of infected babies is 3 years. As with HSV, the infection may be transmitted to the baby at birth; therefore a Caesarean section may be an option.

RUBELLA (GERMAN MEASLES)

This is a virus that is well known to cause fetal abnormality, mainly blindness/cataracts, mental retardation, heart defects, and deafness. These problems only arise, however, if the mother becomes infected *during* pregnancy. Happily, infection is now uncommon because most pregnant women have either had the virus in the past and are immune, or have been vaccinated against it. This vaccination programme has resulted in a dramatic decrease in cases of rubella among pregnant women. In a few cases, vaccination does not provide complete protection from infection, so the rubella blood test is usually one of the first performed at the antenatal clinic. If your test shows that you are not immune and during pregnancy you come in contact with someone (usually a child) who has the symptoms, or develop a flu-like illness yourself, another blood test can be done. If you become infected after week 16 of pregnancy, the baby is very unlikely to be affected. If infection occurs between 12 and 16 weeks, there is a 50 per cent chance that the infection will be passed on to the baby, but only 50 per cent of these babies are affected, mainly by varying degrees of deafness. If infection occurs before week 12 of pregnancy, there is about an 80 per cent chance that the baby will be infected, and an 80 per cent chance that it will have serious abnormalities of the eyes, brain, and heart. Some mothers may choose to have a termination in this case, but it is possible to have a fetal blood sample (see Chapter 4) to tell whether the infection has been passed to the baby. The advantage of this is that the baby may be among the 20 per cent not infected; if the test does confirm the infection and the parents choose termination, it is carried out that much later.

SYPHILIS

Syphilis is caused by a parasite and is transmitted sexually, but the advent of penicillin treatment has resulted in a dramatic reduction in the numbers of cases of this disease. The course of the disease may stretch over a long period, beginning with genital ulcers and going through several stages. The Wassermann test is done in the antenatal clinic to check for syphilis infection. Later blood tests that measure antibodies can give a definitive prenatal diagnosis of infection.

## TOXOPLASMOSIS

This infection is caused by a parasite that is commonly found in cats, who usually pick up the disease by eating infected animals and excrete the parasite's eggs in their faeces. Infected cats show no symptoms. The incidence of the disease varies greatly between countries, and depends partly on meat handling practices. It is much more common in continental Europe than in the US and the UK. As with CMV, infected mothers usually show no symptoms but the infection can be transmitted to the baby in up to 60 per cent of cases. Infection can result mainly in abnormalities of the brain and growth retardation. The chance that infection will be passed on to the baby and that the baby will be affected, depends on the stage of pregnancy when infection occurs. Both the risk of transmission and damage are highest if infection occurs during the first trimester. Prompt diagnosis and treatment of the mother with antibiotics has been shown to reduce the risk of damage by about 50 per cent. In mothers with a proven recent infection, detailed ultrasound scans will be performed to check the growth of the baby and the development of its brain, and a fetal blood sample can be taken at 20–22 weeks to check if the infection has definitely been transmitted. In cases where this is confirmed, and no abnormalities can be seen on ultrasound, the majority of babies will be normal. If you decide to continue with the pregnancy, different antibiotics will be prescribed.

To protect yourself from infection, you should not handle cat litter without wearing rubber gloves, you should cook all meat until well done, and wash thoroughly any cooking implements that are used in handling raw meat.

## VAGINAL/URINARY TRACT INFECTIONS

These become more common during pregnancy because of hormonal changes. They are not known to have any effect on the baby. However, if you develop a serious infection or illness as a result of a urinary tract infection, you should tell your doctor because the risks of prematurity and miscarriage are increased. There is one particularly dangerous vaginal infection – beta haemolytic streptococcus – that can cause serious, even lethal pneumonia in the baby. If this infection has been identified in a previous pregnancy, then you should be tested to see if the organism is still present. If it is, the risk to the baby can be reduced by taking antibiotics. A Caesarean section may be an option to consider.

## MULTIFACTORIAL CONDITIONS

These are caused by the interactions of a number of different factors, both genetic and environmental. Neural tube defects such as spina bifida and anencephaly, which affect the developing fetal central nervous system, are good examples of this. These occur most frequently in Celtic populations: the highest frequency in the world is found among the Irish, both in Eire and Northern Ireland, but the next highest frequency occurs in the valleys of south Wales and on the west coast of Scotland. A woman who has had one child with a neural tube defect has about a 5 per cent chance of having another affected child, although the defect may be different next time. For example, the first baby may be born with spina bifida and the second with anencephaly. In the past, the frequencies with which these defects occurred varied from year to year, leading people to look for causes in anything from diets to weather. It has recently been shown that the chance of having recurrent neural tube defects (such as spina bifida and anencephaly) can be reduced by taking vitamins and folic acid just before the mother becomes pregnant and in the early stages of the pregnancy. This is because folic acid seems to be essential for proper development of the nervous system.

Heart defects and cleft lip and palate are also considered to be multi-factorial. The causes and therefore recurrence risks of such conditions can be very difficult to determine. The same condition may have several causes, some genetic, some environmental, some a combination of both. Microcephaly ('small head') is an example of this and results when the brain does not grow properly. This may be due to exposure to a terato-gen such as alcohol or X-rays, or it may be associated with a genetic syndrome. Heart defects are often associated with Down syndrome, but can also be the result of infections, drugs, or diabetes in the mother.

You should be aware that many doctors will be at a loss to assign a cause to such conditions. Since the recurrence risk depends entirely on the cause, you may feel very uneasy about embarking on another preg-nancy 'in the dark' later on. In the absence of anything precise, doctors often quote a recurrence risk of 2–5 per cent in such situations. This figure is actually the average of the risk for a genetically based con-dition, and the risk from environmental factors alone, and thus is not very meaningful. If all the known teratogens can be ruled out, then it is likely that the abnormality has a genetic basis, either inherited or a new mutation. Unless there is a family history of the condition, it is unlikely that the cause will be identified. On a more hopeful note, a huge amount of progress has been made in the understanding of genetic disease, which helps in understanding recurrence risks.

## PREGNANCY COMPLICATIONS AND ACCIDENTS IN LABOUR

These can also result in physical abnormalities and mental retardation. All of the screening test results may be well into the normal range, there is nothing to presage any problems, and then something goes wrong at a late stage such as premature labour or pre-eclampsia/toxaemia. Very premature babies can now be sustained, but they are not really ready for life outside the womb because many of their organs are not fully developed. The medical support systems are not the same as those provided in the womb, and things can go wrong. For example, premature babies need oxygen-rich air, but it is now known that treatment with too much oxygen in the incubator can result in blindness in some very premature babies. On the other hand, the baby may be deprived of oxygen during labour or delivery, which can also cause brain damage. Often there are no predictive factors for such events, but there is a large amount of accumulated medical knowledge and experience for dealing with them. This is why fetal monitoring can be so useful, because it enables doctors to identify babies in distress so that immediate treatment can be given.

# 4
# Prenatal testing: screening and diagnosis

## MAIN POINTS

- *Most abnormalities happen in families with no history of the condition.*
- *Screening tests are designed to identify pregnancies at higher than average risk of abnormality.*
- *Diagnostic tests are used to check for specific conditions where there is a known risk factor or abnormal screening test result.*
- *Sometimes several different tests, or repeated tests, are needed to obtain a diagnosis.*
- *Invasive diagnostic tests have some risk for the baby.*
- *Hospitals differ in the tests and expertise available.*

More than 90 per cent of babies with a major disorder are born to parents who have not had themselves, or in their family, any children affected by the condition in question. Therefore, if tests were restricted to those who knew they were at risk, or could be identified as being at risk because of their family or other history, less than 10 per cent of congenital abnormalities would be detected. For this reason, a series of tests are given to all women to 'screen' out those at higher risk for having a baby with an abnormality from those at lower risk.

Screening tests do not diagnose abnormalities; to do so requires the use of 'diagnostic tests'. Only those women who have had abnormal screening test results, or who can otherwise be identified as being at higher risk, will usually be offered diagnostic testing. It is important to realize that most women with a 'positive' screening test will actually be found to have a normal baby when the diagnostic test is carried out later. Unfortunately, it must also be said that, when a screening test is negative, this does not guarantee that the baby will be normal. Screening tests only give an idea of relative risk.

If you have been given a positive screening test result, you will be justifiably anxious, and this feeling may not go away even after you have a negative diagnostic test result. By the time you get this result, you may have convinced yourself that the baby is abnormal.

**Remember: the odds are in your favour for the diagnostic test to show that the baby is not affected by the condition suggested by the screening test.**

Diagnostic tests are more costly and time-consuming to perform than screening tests and, except for ultrasound, carry a risk of miscarriage. Amniocentesis, chorion villus sampling, fetal blood sampling, and fetal skin biopsy (see below) are known as 'invasive' tests because it is necessary to 'invade' the baby's environment in order to perform these tests. Some people would choose to have invasive tests for reassurance, despite the possibility that the test itself carries some risk for the pregnancy. An amniocentesis result that rules out Down syndrome and other chromosome abnormalities is reassuring, but mental disability can occur for a variety of other reasons that have no chromosomal signs. A negative result from one test does not exclude other problems.

Testing provides information for parents and the medical staff caring for them, and the benefits of gaining the information have to be weighed against the risks of obtaining it, especially in the case of invasive testing. The size of the risk and the reliability of the results from invasive tests depend to a large degree on the skill and experience of the people performing and analysing the samples. The risks quoted below are those associated with optimal conditions in centres with a high degree of expertise.

Statistics aside, the *perception* of risk varies widely. Many people have a natural aversion to needles and hospitals and would rather avoid the issue altogether. The idea of an invasive test such as amniocentesis can seem very frightening if the chance of having an abnormal baby seems small. On the other hand, the thought of a late termination, which is mentally and physically very stressful, or a seriously disabled baby, can make an early test seem like a good idea. This is despite the fact that the risk associated with the early test may be greater than the chance that the baby will be affected.

All testing carries another, less obvious risk: the risk that the test will turn up a problem. If this happens, several difficult and painful issues will arise, including attitudes to disability and to abortion. Some people are much happier not knowing, or they may feel that prenatal testing is wrong for religious or ethical reasons. If they are afraid to know, or feel it is wrong to know, they will choose not to 'risk' testing. This is every parent's right. You may also choose to limit the amount and type of testing. If you have decided to continue with the pregnancy under any circumstances, you may wish to have a non-invasive test such as an ultrasound scan to inform you of certain abnormalities so that you have an earlier idea of what care, support, or special services will be needed.

## SCREENING TESTS

There are three main types of screening test:

(1) asking a series of questions to determine the family and mother's 'history' of disease, and other risk factors such as the mother's age;

(2) testing the mother's blood (for signs of infections or abnormal levels of certain chemicals);

(3) ultrasound scanning.

### *The history*

To determine if you are at high risk for having a baby with an abnormality, you will be asked a series of questions at the antenatal clinic.

1. How old are you? Chromosome abnormalities occur more frequently in older mothers, usually taken as those over 35 years old.

2. To which ethnic group do you and your partner belong? This is important because some groups have an increased risk of certain genetic diseases: cystic fibrosis for Caucasians, Tay–Sachs disease in Ashkenazi Jews, sickle cell disease for those of Afro-Caribbean origin, alpha/beta thalassaemia in people from Mediterranean and Asian origin, and neural tube defects for Celtic populations.

3. Is there a family history of inherited disease? For example, if any of your mother's male relatives have haemophilia, you may be a carrier and would be offered testing to check this.

4. What were the outcomes of any previous pregnancies? If any of your children were affected by abnormalities in the past it is important to try to establish the recurrence risk for the current pregnancy.

5. Do you personally have any history of disease? Are you taking any medication for it? For women with diabetes and epilepsy, for example, the risk of abnormality is increased, and certain special tests will be needed to check the baby's condition. Some drug regimes

may need to be changed or the dose monitored while you are pregnant (see Chapter 3).

6. What is your present occupation and that of your partner? This is asked because some people are exposed to teratogens or other risks in the course of their jobs.

7. Do you have any habits that could affect the health of the baby – specifically smoking, drinking, or taking non-prescription drugs?

8. What contraception were you using? This is important for calculating the gestational age of the baby, around which the screening test schedule will be planned.

These questions are asked to identify any risks in your pregnancy, and to determine whether any precautions or special tests are necessary. They constitute in effect the 'first line' of screening. In addition to these questions, your height and weight will be measured, your heart and blood pressure checked, and an internal examination will be performed. You will also be asked for a urine sample, which will be tested for protein, sugar, and ketones, which indicate the health of your kidneys and signs of diabetes. These procedures fall under 'routine pregnancy management' and are of value for monitoring the health of mother and baby.

## Maternal blood tests

At your first visit to the antenatal clinic a blood sample will be taken routinely to test for syphilis, evidence of rubella infection, rhesus antibodies/blood group, and to check the haemoglobin level. Your blood may also be tested for antibodies to HIV, the virus associated with AIDS. Other blood tests will be carried out routinely, and you may not be informed of them at the time.

AFP (ALPHA-FETOPROTEIN)
*Why is it done?*
Alpha-fetoprotein (AFP) is only present in the blood of pregnant women because it is produced by a developing baby. It is the 'alpha' or first protein produced. Therefore it is not found in women who are not pregnant except in very rare diseases such as cancer of the liver. During pregnancy, a small amount of the AFP produced by the baby normally escapes into the mother's circulation. If the nervous system does not develop properly, blood vessels in the spine or brain are exposed, which is why these abnormalities are known as 'neural tube defects'. Large amounts of AFP pass into the amniotic fluid, and from there into the

mother's circulation. For this reason, the level of AFP in the mother's blood is measured to discover if the baby has an open neural tube defect such as anencephaly or spina bifida, or other abnormality linked with higher levels of AFP.

*How is it done?*
A small sample of blood is taken from a vein in the mother's arm and sent to a laboratory for analysis.

*When is it done?*
The best time to measure this is when the baby is 15–17 weeks of gestation.

*What are the risks?*
None.

*What do the results mean?*
It should not be assumed that a high or low AFP level definitely means that the baby is abnormal; further tests are needed to ascertain this, and in many cases the baby may be indeed normal and something else is responsible for the abnormal reading. Overall, about 1 in 30 women have a 'high' AFP result. Although most babies with anencephaly occur when there are high levels of AFP in the mother's blood, some mothers with perfectly normal babies will also have high levels. This can happen if, for example, the placenta is especially leaky, which makes the AFP level in the mother's blood look higher than normal. It may also happen that, in a very small mother, the normal amount of AFP from the baby will seem large because it is more concentrated, less diluted by the mother's blood. One can imagine that a drop of ink in a swimming pool is less concentrated than that same drop in a cup of water, so there would appear to be more ink in the cup. The level of AFP may also be high when there is more than one baby (twins will produce twice as much AFP as one baby). Finally, it may simply be a matter of confusion over dates. A baby that is either older or younger than calculated will produce more or less AFP than predicted.

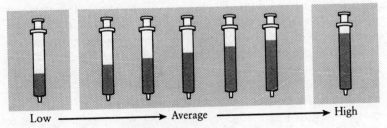

Low ⟶ Average ⟶ High

Range of AFP/triple test results.

The important thing to remember about the AFP screening test is that the 'normal' and 'abnormal' ranges overlap quite a bit. In general, 1 in 15 babies where the level is 'high' will actually have spina bifida or anencephaly, while about 1 in 2000 babies will have spina bifida when the level is 'normal'. You can still have a baby with spina bifida when the level is 'normal' and you can still have a normal baby when the level is 'high'. Women with a 'high' level of AFP in their blood should be offered a detailed ultrasound scan to look for evidence of neural tube defects. In some centres, an amniocentesis is offered to measure the level of AFP in the amniotic fluid.

## MATERNAL BLOOD SCREENING FOR DOWN SYNDROME

This is also known as the 'triple test'. In the last few years, it has been realized that the levels of certain chemicals in the blood of some mothers carrying Down syndrome babies may be different from those in mothers carrying babies unaffected by the syndrome. These babies tend to be smaller and produce less AFP so the amount in the mother's blood is less. This result, combined with an **above average** level of human chorionic gonadotrophin (HCG, the hormone produced by the placenta that is used in home pregnancy tests), and a **below average** level of oestriol (a normal pregnancy hormone) indicate an increased risk of having a Down syndrome baby.

*When is it done?*

This test is done at about 16 weeks on the same blood sample as the AFP test where it is offered. There is a lot of research going on in this field and it is possible that in the near future the test or a variant of it will be refined to work just as well at 12 weeks.

*What do the results mean?*

Because this is a screening test, it will not tell you if your baby has or does not have Down syndrome – it will only provide an expression of the risk. The result is often given as 'screen positive' or 'screen negative', depending on whether the risk is above or below 1 in 280. From then on, it should be your decision whether or not to go ahead and have an amniocentesis to determine if the baby is definitely affected. Some people may feel that a risk of 1 in 100 is reassuringly low; others may feel that the risk of even 1 in 1000 is too high. It all depends on your personal point of view. How important is it for you to know for sure if the baby has Down syndrome? Are you willing to accept an increased risk of miscarriage in order to find out?

Since this is a screening test, you need to remember the same things about these results as for high AFP results: many women with 'abnormally' low levels of AFP have normal babies and mothers who have an AFP level in the normal range may have Down syndrome babies. This is because the 'abnormal' and 'normal' ranges overlap quite a bit and other things – such as the size of the baby, whether the mother has diabetes, and whether the dates are right – can confuse the results.

## Ultrasound

### Why is it done?

Ultrasound can be used to detect structural abnormalities that may be small (cleft lip) or large (missing limbs), but it cannot detect genetic abnormalities that have no structural features such as haemophilia.

Screening is usually performed at around 20 weeks, by a radiographer or obstetrician, but an additional scan is now commonly offered at 12 weeks. The main purpose of the early scan is to check how advanced the pregnancy is, how many babies there are, if they are alive, if they are growing properly, and if there are any major abnormalities. Recently, it has been noticed that most fetuses with serious chromosome abnormalities have extra fluid behind the neck, which can be detected by ultrasound at this stage of pregnancy.

At the 20-week scan, the position of the placenta and the amount of amniotic fluid are checked. The purpose of this scan is to examine the baby thoroughly to pick up both large and small abnormalities. However, differences in the standards of equipment and skill of operators mean that this ideal is not always achieved in routine practice. If something suspicious is picked up during ultrasound screening, or when the parents are known to be at high risk for a specific abnormality, then a detailed 'diagnostic' scan is carried out by an expert.

To summarize, as a screening test, ultrasound is used to provide an overall picture of the baby's condition; as a diagnostic tool, it is used to look for signs of a specific abnormality. For example, if another screening test result such as high AFP suggests that the baby might have spina bifida, ultrasound will be used by an expert in a diagnostic capacity. Similarly, if the fetal heart looks unusual during the routine scan, a detailed scan carried out by a heart specialist will help define if indeed the heart is abnormal and the precise nature of the condition.

### How is it done?

Ultrasound works by bouncing high-frequency sound waves, produced by an ultrasound transducer or probe, through the mother's tissues to the baby, placenta, and amniotic fluid surrounding the baby. Every tissue, in both the mother and the baby, has a slightly different density, and they each reflect the sound waves back in a slightly different way. They are received by the transducer, which builds up a picture of the tissues being scanned with the help of a computer. Modern ultrasound technology has been refined so that the sound pulses are only 1 microsecond long (one-millionth of a second), followed by a millisecond of silence (one-thousandth of a second).

The scan is done by covering part of the mother's abdomen with oil or jelly on which the probe glides. The figure below shows a head in profile, the face uppermost.

Some centres use the technique of vaginal scanning, in which the probe is inserted into the vagina instead of gliding over the abdomen. This can show quite a lot of detail about the baby in early pregnancy, although only the most major deformities will be visible at this stage. A full bladder is not required; the insertion of the probe is similar to an internal examination. As a scanning method early on it offers excellent pictures of the baby.

*What are the risks?*

None are known, for either abdominal or vaginal methods. The Royal College of Obstetricians and Gynaecologists of Great Britain and the American National Institutes of Health have both published studies in which no adverse effects were found. This is an important advantage of ultrasound over other diagnostic tests because it is the only one that is not invasive.

*What do the results mean?*

A skilled operator will be able to see if there are any defects in the heart, lungs, brain, head, spine, kidneys and bladder, digestive system, and limbs. When an abnormality is picked up by ultrasound, it is important to find out if it is confirmed by other test results or repeated scans. If

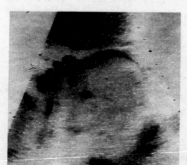 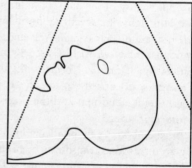

Ultrasound image of a baby's head in profile.

so, the next thing to find out is if this is the only problem or whether there are additional abnormalities. Next, the severity of the abnormality must be determined. For example, in some cases of a cleft lip and palate, there are other defects in the brain, heart, kidneys, and hands; the common link may be a serious chromosomal abnormality such as trisomy 13.

If there are no other defects, the size and type of the cleft (only lip or also palate) should be determined, as this influences the effects on the baby and the kind of operation that the baby will need after birth. If only the lip is affected, only one operation is usually needed for what is a relatively simple repair. When the palate is affected, and the defect is large, several operations may be necessary. In addition, in severe cases parents need to be aware of possible problems with feeding and speech.

This is a testing method where a lot depends on the skill and experience of the operator and the stage at which the scan is done. Small abnormalities can be difficult to see early on, but become more obvious later in pregnancy. However, even experienced people can 'see' abnormalities that are not really there because some images are very difficult to interpret; sometimes the baby is in a difficult position for scanning, or keeps moving. Likewise, it is possible to miss things on a scan. The results of a scan are considered in combination with other test results and, if necessary, these tests can be repeated.

In some centres the person doing the scan is not allowed to tell the parents the results. This is because it is sometimes necessary to discuss the results with an obstetrician to ensure that they are interpreted correctly.

## BETWEEN SCREENING AND DIAGNOSIS

If you get an abnormal screening test result, it is your choice whether or not to have further testing. Diagnostic tests, with the exception of ultrasound, do carry a risk for the baby. It is true, however, that women with normal babies who have this confirmed by a diagnostic test such as amniocentesis feel less anxious during the rest of the pregnancy and after than those who decide against further testing. Those who do have an abnormality detected by a diagnostic test can then choose whether or not to terminate the pregnancy.

Positive routine screening tests early in pregnancy can be very upsetting and worrying for parents. It is often necessary to wait several weeks before diagnostic testing can be carried out and the results known. An important point to bear in mind is that the majority of positive screening test results are 'false positive results' and the baby is not actually affected. Even once you have accepted this, it can be very difficult to get rid of the idea that something is wrong with the baby after the possibility has been raised. Even when you get a normal diagnostic test result, you may have nagging doubts and suspicions about the accuracy of the test, whether you are being told everything, and whether the baby might have other abnormalities that require other tests. When you feel extremely anxious, your mind tends to focus on thoughts that make you feel more anxious. You can become caught up in a spiral of increasing worry while other people – medical staff, partner, relatives – may not appreciate how you feel. The medical staff will have seen with their own eyes that most babies with abnormal screening test results are normal. Your partner's and relatives' different perspectives may allow them to feel greater reassurance when told that the baby is most likely to be unaffected, especially once a diagnostic test shows this to be the case.

It does not help that practitioners and expectant parents can have different priorities when it comes to relaying test results. In some places, the policy is that only positive results are relayed, the 'no news is good news' approach. This should be clarified by your doctor, as well as how (letter, phone call, visit) and by whom (doctor, nurse) the news will be delivered. In any case, you should be informed of the approximate date of the test results; if this passes without any news, you should get in touch with the doctor or clinic.

## DIAGNOSTIC TESTS

### Amniocentesis

#### Why is it done?

Amniocentesis is a diagnostic test performed to check for chromosome disorders, for other genetic disorders, and sometimes if the level of AFP is high. It is most widely used for older mothers, those who have had a previous baby with a chromosome abnormality, and when the triple test result suggests a high risk of Down syndrome. Amniocentesis can also be used to check for a wide range of inherited diseases such as Tay–Sachs disease and cystic fibrosis where there is a known risk factor such as a family history. In some centres, amniocentesis is done if the AFP level is high to check for evidence of a neural tube defect like spina bifida. However, in many centres it is now possible to provide a definitive diagnosis using ultrasound to look at the baby's head and spine, without the need for an amniocentesis.

*How is it done?*

An ultrasound scanner is used to locate the baby, the placenta, and the best place from which to take a sample of the amniotic fluid. The mother's abdomen is then washed with an antiseptic solution; a local anaesthetic is used in some centres. Guided by the ultrasound image, the doctor inserts the sampling needle through the abdomen, into the womb to remove some fluid from around the baby, making sure to avoid the baby and the placenta.

It is natural to feel anxious about this, but the feeling is like having a blood sample taken from your arm and it does not take very long. Afterwards, you will usually be asked to rest for a little while and take things easy for the next couple of days. During this time, you may feel tenderness where the needle was inserted. It is not uncommon to lose small amounts of clear fluid from the vagina, but if you are bleeding, feeling pain, or running a temperature, you must see your doctor immediately.

The pale yellow amniotic fluid contains some of the baby's cells, which have shed naturally. The sample is sent to the laboratory, where the cells will be encouraged to grow and divide (cultured) for about 10–14 days. When there are sufficient cells, a special chemical is added to the culture that 'freezes' the cells in the middle of division, at just the right stage for their chromosomes to be counted and analysed. This is what is known as 'karyotyping'. For the diagnosis of inherited diseases, the DNA from the cells is examined using specific tests to determine if the genes are normal or abnormal.

*When is it done?*

Amniocentesis is usually done at 16 weeks. Although recently it has been done at around 10–13 weeks, the risks are higher.

*What are the risks?*

The risk of miscarriage through the amniocentesis procedure is about 1 in 100. Although there are a few reports of damage caused to the baby by the needle during amniocentesis, this should not happen if ultrasound is used to monitor continuously the position of the needle.

*What do the results mean?*

If there is a problem with the baby's chromosomes, the answer may be very simple (too many, too few) or very complex (pieces missing, translocated, stuck together). Chromosome disorders are extremely variable in their effects, from no symptoms at all to major physical and/or mental disability and everything in between. Depending on the type of problem, the doctor may be able to give you a diagnosis of a well-known syndrome like Down, or may have to say honestly, 'I don't know'. Occasionally you and your partner will be asked to give a blood sample to check your chromosomes. If one of you has *exactly* the same 'abnormality' then, like you, the baby is likely to be normal.

Results from an amniocentesis are usually not available for 2–3 weeks for chromosome studies. This is the same for most types of metabolic disease (enzyme analysis). In the case of DNA testing, the results take about 1–2 weeks or less with new methods. If the test is being done because of a suspected neural tube defect, the results will be available in 3–4 days.

Re-testing is sometimes necessary if there is not enough fluid obtained or if the cells do not grow properly. In a small number of cases, the result may be uncertain because there is a mixture of normal and abnormal cells, known as 'mosaicism'.

## Chorion villus sampling (CVS)

### Why is it done?

CVS is carried out for the same reasons as amniocentesis; that is, to check for chromosome abnormalities and to diagnose inherited disorders. It is not used to check for suspected neural tube defects. The placenta is formed from the same cells as the baby, so it is generally true that if the cells from the placenta are normal, so is the baby. The main advantage of CVS is that it is usually done earlier in pregnancy than amniocentesis, and a diagnosis should be possible in theory by 12 weeks of gestation. The disadvantage is that it is a newer technique, which means that its track record for safety and accuracy is not as well established as for amniocentesis, and there are fewer doctors with expert knowledge.

### How is it done?

CVS is carried out on a small sample of placental material (chorionic villi). CVS is done transabdominally (through the mother's abdomen, as in amniocentesis) or transcervically (through the cervix). Transabdominal CVS is similar to amniocentesis in that it is performed with a needle through the mother's abdomen, taking a sample of the villi rather than the amniotic fluid. In transcervical CVS, a thin catheter is passed into the vagina and through the cervix to collect the villi. In the traditional feet-in-stirrups position, a vaginal speculum (the metal instrument familiar from internal examinations) is inserted, through which the catheter is passed under ultrasound guidance. This is similar to having a cervical smear or an IUD (contraceptive coil) inserted. The feeling is usually discomfort rather than pain, but some women do feel pain. The whole thing lasts only a few minutes.

The advice post-amniocentesis applies for post-CVS – take it easy for a couple of days and report any bleeding, tenderness, or temperature immediately.

*When is it done?*

CVS is usually done after 10 weeks because there is a suggestion that abnormalities of the feet and hands can occur if it is done earlier.

*What are the risks?/What do the results mean?*

When CVS was first introduced it undoubtedly offered advantages because it could be done at an early stage. There are, however, conflicting reports as to its safety and accuracy. Some studies suggest that it is just as safe as amniocentesis; other reports have indicated that the risks of miscarriage and of getting a false result are higher with CVS. The problems reported vary widely between centres and the true picture is still unclear.

As with amniocentesis, re-testing is sometimes necessary if the cells do not grow or the result is uncertain. A further problem with CVS is that sometimes the sample is contaminated by the mother's cells. Mosaicism is also more common with CVS because of the nature of the placenta itself: cells taken from the placenta do not always match genetically those of the baby. There may be a mixture of cells found in the sample. Then the question arises as to which is truly representative of the baby's condition. Most of these cases can now be sorted out by further testing.

## Other special techniques

FETAL BLOOD SAMPLING (FBS)

*Why is it done?*

In some circumstances, it is necessary to analyse a sample of the baby's blood for diagnosis. This technique is also called cordocentesis because it involves taking a blood sample from the umbilical cord. FBS can be used if an abnormality with a likely chromosomal cause is detected by ultrasound late in pregnancy. It could also be offered if a mother has miscalculated her dates and is found to be at risk for a major genetic disorder late in pregnancy. There are also some conditions such as infections and anaemia where the baby's blood needs to be tested to obtain a diagnosis. Whereas amniocentesis results for chromosome abnormality can take 2–3 weeks, results from FBS for these conditions can be obtained in 3–4 days. FBS is a specialist technique, however, and the necessary skills and experience are found only in a few centres.

*How is it done?*

It is very similar to amniocentesis and transabdominal CVS, and sometimes even quicker. The place where the umbilical cord joins the placenta is visualized using ultrasound. A fine needle is passed through the mother's abdomen and into the cord and a small blood sample is taken. The results usually only take a few days.

*When is it done?*

FBS is usually carried out after 20 weeks.

*What are the risks?*

In the specialist centres where this is done, the risk of miscarriage is 1 or 2 in 100, which is similar to that for amniocentesis and CVS. If it is done earlier than 20 weeks the risks are higher.

*What do the results mean?*

This depends on why the test was carried out. In the case of chromosome abnormalities and inherited diseases, the information is the same as that obtained through amniocentesis or CVS. When FBS is done for infections such as rubella and toxoplasmosis, the result will tell you whether or not the baby has the infection, not whether the baby developed any abnormalities as a result of the infection. In women with

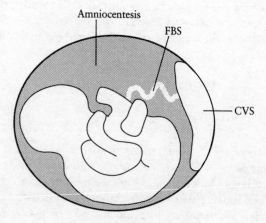

Amniocentesis, CVS, and FBS.

**Table 4.1** Diagnostic tests

| Test* | What it can detect | When it is done |
|---|---|---|
| Ultrasound | Structural defects such as spina bifida and small defects associated with chromosome abnormalities<br><br>Genetic syndromes<br>Growth abnormalities<br>Multiple pregnancies | 10 weeks–term |
| Amniocentesis | Chromosome disorders<br>Infections<br>Single gene disorders<br>Metabolic disorders | 16–18 weeks |
| CVS | Chromosome disorders<br>Single gene disorders<br>Metabolic disorders<br>Infections | transcervical 10–12 weeks<br>transabdominal<br>10 weeks–term |
| FBS | Chromosome disorders<br>Metabolic disorders<br>Single gene disorders<br>Infections<br>Blood disorders (clotting, rhesus)<br>Placental problems (for example, lack of oxygen) | 20 weeks–term |
| FSB | Inherited skin disorders | 15–22 weeks |

* CVS, chorion villus sampling; FBS, fetal blood sampling; FSB, fetal skin biopsy.

rhesus disease, the test is done to assess the baby's anaemia, and whether a blood transfusion is necessary.

FETAL SKIN BIOPSY (FSB)
*Why is it done?*
This technique is only used to detect serious genetic skin disorders where there is a family history, such as epidermolysis bullosa lethalis (EBL) where the skin layers do not attach properly to each other, causing

terrible blistering. Because these conditions are rare, FSB is carried out in very few centres in the world.

*How is it done?*

This is very similar in principle to transabdominal CVS. Under ultrasound guidance, a fine needle is inserted through the mother's abdomen. A pair of biopsy forceps are then passed through the needle, and they are used to take a minute skin sample, usually from the baby's buttock.

*When is it done?*

FSB is usually done at 15 weeks or later.

*What are the risks?*

In specialist centres, the risk of miscarriage is around 1 or 2 in 100, similar to the other invasive tests described above. The mark on the baby where the sample is taken is virtually invisible.

*What do the results mean?*

FSB will give you a definite answer as to whether or not the baby is affected by the skin disorder in question.

The figure on p. 54 summarizes the different places from where samples are taken for amniocentesis, CVS, and FBS. Table 4.1 summarizes the different uses of the diagnostic tests described in this chapter and when they can be done.

# 5
# Your options once the test results are known

## MAIN POINTS

- *If an abnormality is diagnosed, you may have to choose whether or not to continue with the pregnancy.*
- *It is important to think through all the options even if you 'know' what you want to do.*
- *Specialist counselling and support groups can help you decide what is right for you.*
- *This is a very personal and complex decision; everyone is affected in different ways by their own and other people's feelings.*
- *Depending on the type of abnormality and the stage of pregnancy, there are different options for continuing with the pregnancy and having a termination.*
- *Regardless of which choice you make, the experience can have effects which last for a long time.*
- *The type of abnormality and its cause will determine the chance of it happening again in a future pregnancy.*

If you have an abnormal screening test result that is later confirmed by a diagnostic test, it may be necessary for you to decide whether to continue with the pregnancy or have a termination. This is a very difficult and painful decision, which can be made worse by the fact that you may not have much time to decide. The purpose of this chapter is to help you make the best use of whatever time is available by focusing on the questions that you may want to ask once the test results are known.

Even if you feel you already know what you want to do when you are given the diagnosis, we urge you to read also the section dealing with the alternative. This is because people often have second thoughts after the fact and agonize over what might have been. This is less likely to happen if you know that you have thought everything through and gained as much information as possible before making your decision. Looking back on it, there should be fewer self-recriminations of the 'what if' type if you have explored all the 'ifs' beforehand. Another reason for this is that the risk associated with certain conditions, especially structural abnormalities, can change during the pregnancy as more tests are carried out. This may ultimately affect your decision.

## BREAKING THE NEWS

Different hospitals have different policies when it comes to relaying test results and diagnosis. These range from a letter or phone call to a personal discussion with the doctor. People who deliver such news include nurses, health visitors, and general practitioners in addition to doctors in the hospital. Some couples request specifically for one or the other of them to be contacted depending if the news is bad or good.

It is never easy to break bad news to anxious parents, and some doctors counter this by adopting a jolly, staggeringly inappropriate 'Never mind, you can always get pregnant again' or 'Never mind, you have other children' approach. Ideally, the test results should be explained in detail, in private, with a minimum of jargon, and with plenty of time for questions. When parents are given such devastating information, however tactfully, their reactions can vary widely: anger; denial; absolute calm; uncontrolled weeping; or even hysterical laughter. Some people appear very calm in the clinic, partly because they don't want to break down in front of the doctor, but may weep for hours afterwards. You should not be worried if you feel any or all of these things.

After a few hours or more, you may have trouble remembering the details of your conversation with the doctor. Some hospitals provide tape recorders and tapes so that you can take away a record of the conversation to review later. It can also be useful to play the tape for close friends or relatives who want to know 'what the doctor said'. You can also bring your own tape recorder, and you can ask the doctor to write down any details that are not clear.

It is quite likely that the best description of the condition may well seem vague and unhelpful. This is often a true reflection of the state of the understanding in the field. Some chromosome abnormalities are especially difficult to predict, but the degree of disability caused by spina bifida also varies enormously. It is not at all uncommon to find that it is impossible to arrive at a precise description of the effects of the abnormality on the baby.

## COUNSELLING

Once you have been given a diagnosis, an important step in arriving at the right decision for you is counselling with your doctor or genetic counsellor. You can be referred to a genetic counsellor or specialist genetic centre by your general practitioner, obstetrician, or other medical staff. If a referral is not offered and you want more information, you can ask to be referred.

Genetic counselling mainly involves describing the condition as fully as possible, the cause (if known), the way it is inherited, and the risk of recurrence. In every other area of medicine, when we have a problem, we ask the doctors what to do and they tell us, or at least they tell us what they would do in the same situation. This should not happen in genetic counselling – in fact, something is wrong if it does. Some parents report after their initial meetings with these counsellors that they are 'distant' and 'unhelpful'. This is often out of a mistaken belief that the counsellor will tell them what to do, but this is exactly what they are trying *not* to do. It is their job to provide you with the information you need to help you determine the best decision for you. They will help you to think through your options, while keeping their own opinions out of the discussion.

The aim of good counselling is for the parents to realize that the final choice is theirs so that they do not feel that they have been pressured into continuing the pregnancy if they wanted an abortion, or into having an abortion when they wanted to keep the baby. Above all, they should not feel that they have done 'what the doctor wanted us to do'. Neither should it be implied that 'you should not have had the test if you were not prepared to act on the result'. There is no obligation on your part, either to the hospital or to the doctor, to have an abortion if an abnormality is detected. Opting for testing does not in any sense mean that you are tacitly agreeing to terminate the pregnancy if the tests detect an abnormality.

It is true that parents can be influenced by the doctor's or counsellor's own perception and presentation of the information they are being given, especially for the rarer conditions where knowledge and experience are limited. Ideally, the counsellor should outline *all* of the options open to you, and help you to determine which is the best for your situation. This is known as 'non-directive' counselling. It has been argued that truly non-directive counselling is not possible because, if the abnormality is not lethal, the option of abortion is implicit in the offer of counselling. Therefore, you have already been 'directed' to a certain extent by being counselled. The subtlety of this argument may seem irrelevant to many parents but it is an indication of how seriously counsellors take their role.

Aside from formal counselling, support groups are an important source of information and emotional back-up. Unfortunately, it is beyond the scope of this book to provide a comprehensive listing of such groups worldwide. Appendix 3 lists a number of groups in the UK and North America. You can obtain details of groups in your area from your hospital, doctor, clinic, or counsellor; they are also often listed in the telephone directory.

## THINGS YOU MAY WANT TO ASK

There are several important questions for you to consider in making the decision as to whether or not to continue with the pregnancy. Once you have been through them, you will be in a better position to judge which is the best option for you. We do not mean to suggest that this approach will provide a 'formula' for decision-making. (For one thing, the answers to the questions relating to the condition itself may be 'I don't know'.) The questions are there as prompts to help you focus on the practical and emotional issues involved.

- *What are the physical and mental effects associated with the condition?*
- *What length and kind of life would someone with this condition have?*
- *What is the cause?*
- *What is the chance of it happening again?*

Having spoken either with the doctor in the hospital or your own general practitioner, you may wish to get further information from specialists, for example, a plastic surgeon if the baby has a facial cleft; support groups or parents with affected children; teachers or others involved in caring for affected children; other books.

It is also important that you and your partner (if you have one) try to address a series of issues relating to your own personal circumstances. Below are listed some specific questions which expand on the above points and will be applicable to differing degrees depending on the condition.

## The condition itself and its treatment

- What is the physical appearance of the abnormality likely to be? You may wish to see photographs, or meet parents with affected children.

- Can the appearance be improved by surgery or physiotherapy? Is the child likely to suffer during these procedures?

- How much effect would the treatment have on the child's quality of life?

- What degree of physical disability is associated with the abnormality? Will the child be mobile or need assistance? What kind of assistance – cane, crutches, wheelchair? Will the child be totally bedbound?

- Is any sort of prenatal or postnatal surgery or other treatment (drugs, transplant, gene therapy) possible? If so, where?

- What kind of facilities, for example, special schools or physiotherapy, would be needed to care for someone with this condition?

- Are there any other diseases associated with this condition? (For example, many babies with Down syndrome also have heart defects that can affect their survival.)

- Will the effects change – become worse or better – as the child gets older?

- Will the child be able to support and care for itself when you get ill, old, or die?

- Will the child be able to get married and have children?

- What is the life expectancy of someone with the condition?

## Your personal situation

- Do you have a religious or moral objection to abortion on any grounds?

- Do you feel that any sort of disability would be unacceptable?

- Which types of disability could you come to terms with?

- Is the relationship with your partner strong enough to survive raising a disabled child/having an abortion?

- Do you have any other children? If so, how would they be affected by having a disabled child in the family?

- What will your friends, family, and colleagues think if you have a disabled child/abortion? How much does this matter to you?

- *How old are you and your partner? This is important in considering future pregnancies.*

- *Have you had an infertility problem? What are the chances of getting pregnant again?*

- *If you have a partner, can one of you give up work if necessary to care for the child?*

- *Are you a single parent? If so, what are your options if you have to give up work to care for the child?*

- *Can you afford financially the treatment/therapy needed? Would a nurse be needed? Can you afford it?*

- *Does your accommodation need to be modified (wheelchair ramps, etc.)?*

- *Ultimately, are you and your partner in agreement about the option you wish to take?*

## MAKING YOUR DECISION

The decision whether or not to terminate a wanted pregnancy is one of the most traumatic that any parent can ever experience. An especially difficult thing for parents to decide is whether the abnormality diagnosed is 'serious', and how it relates to their personal feelings about disability and abortion. The same condition may be seen as very severe by some people but relatively unimportant or trivial by others. Some parents would look towards therapy or special schooling to maximize the child's chances, but other parents, given the same diagnosis but with different attitudes to disability, would opt for termination right away. Others may feel that the prospects for the child are not that bad but doubt their own ability to cope both with a disabled child, and the judgement of other people. Worries about the termination procedure itself and the potential physical, psychological, and emotional effects will all be factors in making this decision.

For many conditions, the doctor will be unable to describe precisely what physical and/or mental disabilities the baby will have. Sometimes even after all the testing and waiting, you may simply be given another statistical risk. What do you do when you are told that the baby has been infected by rubella, and there is a 50/50 chance that it will be mentally disabled? Do you have a termination when you know that there is a 'good chance' that the baby is normal, or do you carry on with the pregnancy when you know there is a 'high risk' of the baby being seriously disabled?

The thing to keep in mind at all times is this: people react differently to the news that their baby is affected by an 'abnormality' and make different decisions based on the complex mixture of their individual beliefs, background, and feelings. There is no such thing as a 'right' or 'wrong' decision in these situations. After all, often an 'abnormality' is really part of the spectrum of normality, a variation in the *range*. Your perceptions and feelings about the particular variation in question are what matter.

It is not unusual to change your mind several times right up to the moment of termination or birth. Although it is your choice, it may not seem that you have any choice at all; you may feel that you have no control and are being pushed back and forth between two equally unacceptable sets of circumstances. This is another reason for learning as much about the alternative course of action as you can, even if you 'know' what is right for you. Conflicts may arise not only in your own mind but with people who are close to you, such as your partner and family.

## 'WHAT DO OTHER PEOPLE DO?'

Parents often want to know what other people in similar situations have done. However, there is no consistent answer. This is because people can react in completely different ways depending on their particular background, perceptions, and circumstances. Your ideas may well change from day to day or even hour to hour. Many things and people can influence your perceptions and feelings, and it can help to be aware of these different pressures in deciding what is best for you and your partner.

**Doctors** Once the diagnosis is known, you will be on the receiving end of different medical opinions that may conflict with each other. No one is completely neutral, including doctors, whose advice is partly based on the cases that they have dealt with in the past and their own prejudices.

**Friends and family** You may also find opinions being offered by friends and family, who have their own ideas about the condition. A recurring worry for parents is, 'What will my friends/family/colleagues think?'

**Religion and culture** The cultural and religious values held in your community are important influences on your thinking, sometimes embodied forcefully by religious leaders who can exert powerful pressures on people in this situation. It should be said that they can also provide welcome support.

**Society's attitudes relating to abortion and disabled people** The way that personal stories are reported in the media, for example, can make a lasting impression depending on whether the sympathy seems to lie with the mother/parents or the baby. Prenatal testing itself is generally depicted positively in the media, but society takes a paradoxical view of abnormalities; there is a desire to provide a positive environment for affected people, while more and more resources are directed at prevention. Different prejudices operate in different cultures (male versus female children) or within different groups in society.

**Personal experiences** If you have experienced the condition yourself or in your family, your perception of it will be different to that of someone with no family history. In addition, if you have had experience of a mild form of the condition yourself or in your family, your decision may well be different from someone who has experienced or cared for someone with a severe form of the condition.

If the same abnormality has arisen in a previous pregnancy, you may not make the same decision as you did at that time in the past. The experience of the previous pregnancy and changes in your outlook or circumstances may lead you to a different decision.

**Your own feelings about abnormality in general** Many people also have deeply felt convictions about which, if any, abnormalities they could live with in their child. People have very high expectations of their children. Some parents feel that any physical defect, even if it is correctable, is unacceptable; for others, mental impairment would be unbearable, but they could come to terms with a degree of physical disability.

**Relationship with your partner** Given the fact that each person carries around a unique combination of many different influences, it is not surprising that partners can disagree about which option to take. If both partners have strong and opposing views, then one of them will have to go along with the other's wishes. If this is done grudgingly or falsely, bitterness and resentment can further strain a relationship that is already under tremendous pressure. The opposite scenario may also arise. Faced with such a difficult decision, it can be tempting to try to offload the burden of responsibility for making it on to someone else. It may be a relief in the short term to have the decision made for you, but the partner who decides unilaterally will suffer blame and recriminations if the other partner has second thoughts later.

**Welfare of existing children** Many parents manage to balance admirably the needs of a disabled child with those of their unaffected children, but it is not easy. People who have grown up with disabled siblings often resent the disruption to normal family life, and the fact that the needs of the disabled child demand the highest priority. The stress on the parents' financial, emotional, and physical resources can make lasting impressions on the other children, which adds an extra burden of guilt for the parents.

## CASE HISTORIES

- A 31 year-old woman with two normal children came to the antenatal clinic at 16 weeks for a routine AFP test. She forgot all about the test until a week later when she was asked to come to the clinic to discuss the result. The doctor said that the AFP level was considered low and that her risk of having a baby with Down syndrome was 1 in 60. He said that having an amniocentesis would give a definite answer, but that the result would take about 3 weeks to come through. The woman was very upset because the whole situation was so unexpected, she was worried about having an amniocentesis, and did not want to wait so long for an answer; the doctor explained that amniocentesis did carry a risk of miscarriage but that it was necessary to have a sample of the baby's cells to obtain a diagnosis. The cells then needed time to grow before they could get an answer. The woman decided to go ahead with the test, and 3 weeks later was asked to come back to the clinic. The doctor said that the result showed that the baby did not have Down syndrome, but another chromosome abnormality, trisomy 18. He said that the baby would be severely disabled and might die before birth or survive for several months. After discussion with her partner, they decided to have a termination.

- One couple who were both affected by achondroplasia (dwarfism) and worked in a circus came for prenatal diagnosis because their preference was for a child who also had achondroplasia. Their home at the circus had been specially adapted for their stature, which a normal child would outgrow, and they felt that a normal child would not have the same employment prospects with the circus as they had. Although they were distressed to find that their child was 'normal', the parents adjusted to the changes that this meant for their lifestyle and now have a second normal child.

- A 30 year-old teacher of children with special needs came for an amniocentesis because her high AFP level suggested a risk of spina bifida. In addition to measuring the level of AFP in the amniotic fluid a karyotype for chromosome disorders was done. She had a lot of experience teaching children with Down syndrome and interacting with their families, and was prepared to continue with the pregnancy if it were diagnosed. She felt, however, that spina bifida was a severely disabling disease and would choose termination if it were diagnosed. The test showed that the baby had Down syndrome and not spina bifida. She decided to continue with the pregnancy.

- One couple had been having infertility treatment for over 8 years. When they finally did conceive, it was found that the fetus was affected by Klinefelter syndrome (see Chapter 2). The mother was desperate for a child and felt that the prospects appeared good from what the genetic counsellor told her. Her husband, however, came from a family where a lot of importance was placed on having normal, fertile sons to continue the line. He was devastated when he found that the syndrome is characterized by infertility and pronounced breast development. The mother decided to continue with the pregnancy. The couple have separated.

- A 23 year-old woman in her first pregnancy had a detailed ultrasound scan at 18 weeks. The baby appeared to be growing well but the doctor was concerned that the scan showed a nuchal oedema (excess fluid under the skin) at the back of the baby's neck. He told the woman that this was associated with an increased risk of Down syndrome. She discussed the situation with her partner, and they asked for an amniocentesis and the assurance that a termination could be carried out right away if something were wrong. Three weeks later, the result of the amniocentesis was normal, but another scan showed that the excess fluid under the skin of the baby's neck was still there. The couple spoke to several doctors, none of whom could assure them absolutely that the baby was normal. The couple became more and more worried and eventually decided to have a termination.

- One mother was not told of a family history of Lesch–Nyhan syndrome, which results in severe mental handicap, until she was pregnant. Her mother had two severely affected brothers and two severely affected sons, all of whom were in hospitals for the mentally disabled. She warned her pregnant daughter that her husband might leave if he found out about the family history. The daughter told her husband that she was at risk for being a carrier of haemophilia, which has the same inheritance pattern and prenatal tests. She insisted that none of the medical personnel tell her husband of the real risk of Lesch–Nyhan syndrome. It turned out that she was a carrier, her *baby was affected, and she had a termination. Two years later, the husband wanted to try for another baby very badly, but she realized that she would have to go through the whole deception again. She told her husband the truth about the risk of Lesch–Nyhan syndrome. He was very shocked and the relationship went through a difficult time, but they eventually got over the episode.*

*Neither partner felt they could go through with another termination if the baby were affected, so they decided to have pre-implantation diagnosis in the next pregnancy. This technique is only used for a few conditions at present. It involves first fertilizing some of the mother's eggs with the partner's sperm (in vitro fertilization), testing the embryos which result, and only implanting in the mother's uterus those that are not affected by the condition in question. The parents went on a waiting list at a specialist centre and were counselled about the risks and possible outcomes. After having three unaffected embryos implanted, the mother was thrilled to find out that the pregnancy test was positive. However, a few days later she miscarried. Even though they had been warned that the method has only about a 20 per cent success rate, she and her husband decided that the cost and the emotional trauma of disappointment were too much to face again. They have gone onto an adoption waiting list.*

- *One couple had a child with cystic fibrosis who was being treated with physiotherapy, and antibiotics for recurrent chest infections. They asked for prenatal diagnosis of the condition for their next pregnancy because they had decided to have a termination if the baby was affected. They already had another unaffected child whom they felt was suffering from neglect because of all the time and energy spent caring for the other child, and taking him repeatedly to the hospital. The husband had recently lost his job and they felt that their financial situation would not enable them to support another affected child. The results of the CVS showed that the baby was affected and a termination was carried out.*

- *A couple who had lost a child to epidermolysis bullosa lethalis (a rare inherited skin disease) decided to try again because prenatal diagnosis through fetal skin biopsy was possible at 18–19 weeks. Unfortunately, the test showed that the baby was affected and the couple opted for termination, but this lasted nearly 24 hours and was very traumatic. Since they were both carriers for the condition, they decided to go on a waiting list for assisted conception using donor sperm. While they were on the waiting list, they consulted their rabbi who forbade them from having donor sperm on religious grounds. A year later they tried for another pregnancy but this resulted in a miscarriage at 8 weeks. By the time they tried again they were both over 35 and at higher risk for chromosome abnormalities as well as the lethal skin condition. The results of both the skin biopsy and the karyotype were normal, and they have since had another normal baby.*

- *A healthy 18 year-old woman came to the antenatal clinic for the first time at 16 weeks. Her blood test showed a raised level of AFP, which suggested the possibility of spina bifida, and she was called back to the clinic for a detailed ultrasound scan. This showed that the baby had spina bifida. There was no history of any genetic disease either in her or her partner's family, and they had never imagined that they could be at risk for anything. After several tearful sessions with relatives and hospital staff, they decided to continue with the pregnancy and give the baby up for adoption at birth.*

- *A 24 year-old woman in her first pregnancy had some bleeding in the first 14 weeks but this eventually stopped. She had an AFP test at 16 weeks, and the level was found to be low. She was told that an amniocentesis was necessary for a diagnosis but was too worried about the earlier bleeding and risk of miscarriage to go through with it. At 20 weeks she had a detailed ultrasound scan, which showed that the baby was small for its age and there were cysts on the brain ('choroid plexus cysts'). The doctor explained that these cysts are seen in about 25 cases in every 1000 and that they often disappear by 23–24 weeks. If they do not disappear, it can mean that the baby has a chromosome disorder such as trisomy 18. He explained that the cysts alone would give a risk of less than 1 per cent of the baby being affected but, combined with the bleeding and growth retardation, would give a risk of 5 per cent. The two options were to wait to see if the cysts disappeared (and have a cordocentesis at 23–24 weeks if they did not) or have a cordocentesis right away to check the baby's chromosomes. After discussing the situation in detail with her partner and other doctors, the woman decided to have a cordocentesis immediately. The result of this showed that the baby did have trisomy 18 and she chose to have a termination.*

## TIMING

You may feel under pressure to make your decision quickly. This is because the pregnancy is advancing every day and your options become more limited as time passes. Termination also becomes more difficult later in pregnancy and certain options for termination are only available at certain stages of pregnancy. In many places, parents are not told about an abnormal diagnosis until the facilities are available to offer an immediate termination. If you have made up your mind and want everything to be over as quickly as possible, this is a good thing. If, however, you are still deliberating, knowing that these facilities are standing by adds to the feelings of pressure. Although the offer of immediate termination is made out of concern and sympathy, you should be given a full explanation of exactly how much time you have and the time schedule for all the different options. If you are unsure about what to do, even if the diagnosis is made quite late in pregnancy there should be time for you to at least talk to a counsellor, other family members, or someone from a support group.

## CONTINUING WITH THE PREGNANCY

### Non-lethal conditions

If you decide to continue with the pregnancy after an abnormality or condition is diagnosed, attention will turn to what might be needed to maximize the baby's chances. Depending on the severity of the problem, there are three possible scenarios relating to whether any treatment, and what type of treatment, is undertaken and whether or not the timing and method of delivery will be altered.

1. There are many conditions that are detectable prenatally that result in few or no long-term physical or mental effects for the baby. A good example of this is mild hydronephrosis (slight excess of fluid in the kidneys), which is detected on routine ultrasound scans in 2–3 per cent of all pregnancies. In about half of the cases, this will disappear by the time of birth; in the rest, the babies have a slightly increased risk of kidney infection. Provided you are aware of this and any infections are treated promptly, there should be no damage to the kidneys. Therefore, for conditions like this, although the original diagnosis can seem worrying, you can be reassured that the outcome is likely to be good, and the pregnancy is managed as normal. It may, however, be the case that such a condition is an indication of a more serious underlying disorder, so you may be offered further tests to check this.

2. There are some conditions that can be corrected with postnatal surgery. In the case of cleft lip and palate, for example, no prenatal

therapy is involved, nor are different approaches to timing or method of delivery (vaginal or Caesarean) necessary. The timing of the surgery may vary from a few hours to several months after birth, depending on the severity of the cleft and the policy of the individual surgeon. However, other abnormalities need *immediate* postnatal evaluation and treatment, such as an omphalocele (where some of the organs are outside the body), diaphragmatic hernia (where some of the abdominal organs are in the chest), or spina bifida. Babies affected by these conditions need to be delivered in centres with specialist personnel and facilities such as a neonatal intensive care unit and paediatric surgeons. For some conditions it may be better to have a Caesarean rather than a vaginal delivery.

3. For a small number of conditions, prenatal treatment is now possible. The best known example of this is rhesus disease, which can be treated quite successfully by giving blood transfusions to the fetus every few weeks. Thousands of children worldwide have survived thanks to this treatment. Other conditions that have been treated prenatally include hydrocephalus (excessive fluid in the brain), pleural effusions (fluid around the lungs), and obstructive uropathy (blocked urinary system) where the excessive fluid in the body of the baby can be drained through catheters. In a few cases, even prenatal heart surgery has been carried out. It should be stressed that, although all of this is very exciting and receives a lot of media attention, the utility of these techniques is very limited. Often the condition has caused too much damage to be corrected. In other situations, there are other abnormalities in addition to the one that can potentially be corrected. For example, excess fluid around the lungs can be drained successfully. If, however, this fluid was due to a viral infection that also produced meningitis, the baby could have severe brain damage.

The other thing to remember about prenatal treatment is that, because very few cases have been attempted, information about the outcome in terms of survival and long-term handicaps is limited. Thus the basis for parental decisions in these cases is less sound than for more common conditions with a long track record for treatment such as cleft lip and palate. Your hopes may be raised by hearing that treatment might be possible, only to find that, in your baby's case, it might not be possible after all because of the type of condition or lack of resources. Even if it is possible, there is no guarantee that the baby will survive, or survive without disability. This emotional roller coaster ride from elation to despair is exhausting.

However, the prospects for prenatal treatment for different conditions are developing all the time. Bone marrow transplantation and gene therapy are two of the potential new treatments, but both technical and ethical aspects are still being studied. Gene therapy has potential use as a way of correcting some single gene defects. Approval has been given for its use with humans in the US and UK for certain conditions under strict constraints. Its use is restricted at present to 'somatic' cells that cannot be passed from one generation to another as opposed to the 'germ line' cells of egg and sperm. New prospects are very exciting, but you should be aware that all pioneering work has associated disappointments in the early stages. Eventually, experience in these techniques may accumulate to the level where most babies will survive without disability, and parents can be told with a high degree of certainty what the outcome will be.

Once you know the diagnosis and what treatment might be possible, there are several ways in which you can prepare yourselves for life with your baby.

- *You can learn more about the condition from books and from other people who have raised children with the condition.*

- *You can join support groups, again to learn about what to expect, but also to gain valuable emotional reinforcement.*

- *You can discuss further the treatment, when it will be done, and how long you and the baby will need to remain in the hospital.*

- *You can talk to surgeons or other medical personnel who will be treating the baby about other babies they have treated.*

- *You can find out what special care will be needed at home afterwards.*

- *You can talk to friends or relatives about any arrangements needed to care for your other children while you are in hospital or when you first get home.*

## Very serious/lethal conditions

Some parents decide against abortion even when the baby has a very serious abnormality. Although conditions such as anencephaly or absent kidneys are lethal, the baby may survive to term because the mother's body continues to support it. Outside the womb it cannot survive, however, and will die within a few hours of birth. Other conditions such as Edward syndrome (trisomy 18) are also described as lethal but babies may survive for 6 months or longer. This is very agonizing for the parents and for the hospital staff caring for the baby. If Edward syndrome is diagnosed late in pregnancy, most obstetricians try to arrange for a caring and supportive delivery, but their aims are not always clear to the parents. If the baby is likely to die during labour or delivery, it would be cruel to carry out fetal heart monitoring or other 'high tech' procedures that would only increase the parents' anxiety. The parents may feel, however, that the baby is not being given the best chance to survive if their perception of the prognosis is different from that of the obstetrician. The debate about Caesarean section also arises here. If the baby shows any distress in a normal pregnancy, it is usually delivered as soon as possible, most often by Caesarean section. The purpose of this in a normal pregnancy is obviously to give the baby the best chance possible. If, however, the baby has a lethal abnormality, the mother's future health will be the top priority.

If the condition is serious but not lethal, and you do not feel that you could cope, it may be possible to have the baby adopted. Depending on the abnormality involved, there may be agencies who can find parents willing to adopt the baby. If you do not want to keep the baby, the possibility of adoption should be explored as soon as possible.

## TERMINATING THE PREGNANCY

Despite the very wide range of fetal abnormalities and parents' perceptions and circumstances, most people opt for termination when a serious abnormality is diagnosed. Looking back, most people say that they would make the same choice again in the same situation. This does not mean that this is the right thing to do, or that this is the right decision for you; it is simply a statistic and a reflection that this is at present the only method of prevention for most major genetic abnormalities.

There is an important difference between terminating a pregnancy for reasons of abnormality at any stage of pregnancy and losing a baby through miscarriage or lethal abnormality: termination requires an active decision on the part of the parents, which introduces a different type of guilt. Making this decision can call into question deep feelings about life in general – what is morally right, your relationship with your partner, your religion. Yet the fact that it is a deliberate choice may lead other people to assume that you have no regrets. It is not unusual at all to feel ambivalent afterwards and wonder if you did the right thing, especially if the doctor could not give you a precise description of the baby's condition.

A full discussion of the ethics of abortion is beyond the scope of this book; in the context of fetal abnormality, it is only one option for you to consider. Your own feelings about ethics and morality will figure in addition to the practical considerations. If you belong to a religious group, its views will also play a part in your decision. Many religious and social groups disapprove of abortion for reasons of abnormality, and these attitudes may be reflected by some of the staff involved in caring for people who are in this situation.

There is no doubt that strongly held religious beliefs can profoundly influence the decisions of parents in this situation. There is a difference, however, between cases where the parents themselves have these feelings and those in which they are pressured by other people such as family, friends, medical staff, colleagues, or even figures in the media. If you have strong convictions either in favour or against abortion or disability, then the right decision for you is probably fairly clear. If the decision of whether or not to keep the baby is determined wholly or in part by forces that are not in complete harmony with your own feelings, it is likely that the psychological after-effects will be worse. It can be quite difficult to get in touch with these feelings, and to have the courage to be true to them, but it can be done with good counselling.

## Methods of termination

The methods used for termination and the exact timing of the operation vary according to the stage of pregnancy and depend on the regulations and resources in your hospital, and any special factors in your case. Pre- and post-abortion counselling are available in some places but not all. Even experienced professionals may fail to appreciate the importance of such counselling. Obstetricians and geneticists who have been in the situation personally have realized that, no matter how much you know about something in theory, you still need practical help in thinking through the options carefully. You need to understand the reasons for your decision and ensure that *you* feel it is the right one for you in the circumstances. Most people feel guilt and regret in coming to terms with things afterwards, but these feelings are less bitter if you have considered all possibilities. Plus, it helps to have some idea of what to expect both mentally and physically.

The way in which the abortion is carried out and the amount and quality of the support before and after the operation all contribute to the way parents feel about the event afterwards. Many hospitals try to ensure that medical staff involved in terminations for abnormality are supportive of such decisions, but some hospitals deal with only a few cases and do not have experienced staff. You may have contact with staff who have widely differing views and lack knowledge of the specific circumstances of the termination.

If your termination is carried out in a hospital (as opposed to a specialized clinic), the type of termination and the location where it is carried out in the hospital depend on the stage of pregnancy and the doctor's judgement. You may be sent to either the gynaecological ward or the maternity ward, depending on the hospital policy. A small number of hospitals have special wards or rooms. You may feel uncomfortable whether among women who have problems unrelated to yours, or among women who will probably be delivering normal babies. You are unlikely to be offered any choice, but you should be given a side room wherever you go.

Specialist abortion clinics may offer terminations on an out-patient or in-patient basis.

Except for cases diagnosed by CVS, termination for reasons of abnormality in a wanted pregnancy is usually carried out later than for most women who have terminations for non-medical reasons, often at about 18–20 weeks. The decision to have a termination is driven by two completely different sets of circumstances. Medical professionals who relate the experience of non-medical termination to termination for abnormality can be unaware of the need for special counselling and support.

There are two types of termination: 'surgical' and 'medical'. Surgical terminations are done either under general or local anaesthetic and involve physically removing the fetus from the uterus. A medical termination is induced by drugs, either as vaginal pessaries or injection. It takes several hours and involves going through labour. We will describe the different methods which may be used. The policies of different hospitals in different regions may mean that very few methods (and sometimes only one) are available.

EARLY SURGICAL TERMINATION
This type of termination is usually performed up to 13 weeks, and would only be offered for those who have had early testing by CVS or other tests. It is carried out in Britain under general anaesthetic. In other countries, including the US, it is done on an out-patient basis in some clinics under local anaesthetic. With a general anaesthetic you are unconscious and wake up when it is all over; with a local anaesthetic, you

are awake and aware of what is going on, but you do not suffer the after-effects of a general anaesthetic.

First, the cervix is dilated and then the fetus is removed from the uterus, as for a D and C (dilation and curettage), all of which takes about 5-10 minutes. If you have had a general anaesthetic you may be asked to stay in the clinic overnight, or at least wait several hours before going home. If you have been given a local anaesthetic you will probably be expected to leave sooner.

There will be no baby for you to see afterwards, but it may be possible to obtain a photo that was taken from the ultrasound screen if you wish to have one.

## LATE SURGICAL TERMINATION

A few obstetricians with specialist experience can perform suction terminations (D and E for dilation and evacuation) up to 24 weeks. This is also done under a general anaesthetic. The advantage of this method is that the mother does not have to go through labour. The disadvantage is that it is difficult to perform post-mortem diagnoses, which might be important if the prenatal diagnosis was uncertain.

## MEDICAL TERMINATION/EARLY INDUCTION OF LABOUR

Many people will have heard of RU 486, the so-called 'abortion pill'. It is used at present up to 10 weeks of pregnancy, before the stage when most abnormalities can be diagnosed, but trials are being conducted to test its use for later abortions.

Later in pregnancy, labour is induced with prostaglandins, drugs that make the womb contract. Prostaglandins are given as vaginal pessaries, or as an injection like an amniocentesis, depending on the doctor's practice. Soon afterwards, contractions start and labour begins. This can be long and painful, lasting anywhere from 6 to 24 hours, or even longer. Pain relief will differ between wards. There is no need for you to suffer; if the pain is too much, ask for help.

The baby is delivered in a similar way to a delivery at term, and sometimes a D and C is needed afterwards to remove any of the placenta that has remained behind.

Many centres now acknowledge the parents' need to see and hold the baby, to give it a name, have a photograph and a funeral. Some parents are so afraid that the baby is a 'monster' that they will have nightmares if they see it. Contact with the baby, even if it is painful, can help the

grieving process. Even for severe abnormalities, in most cases supportive and sympathetic staff will make special efforts to present the baby
very carefully, which actually allays the parents' fears.

## After-effects of termination

After a surgical termination, most women get cramps like a painful
period and some vaginal bleeding may persist for several days or longer.
If the termination was done in late pregnancy, there may be breast
tenderness and milk production. It can take 5–6 weeks before men-
struation resumes and it is important to use a contraceptive if you do not
want to become pregnant again right away.

All terminations, even those carried out early in pregnancy, are
physically shocking for the body. The brain alters hormone levels from
the start of pregnancy and takes a while to realize that there is no longer
a baby before restoring them to normal. Thus you may still feel pregnant for days or longer after the termination. One common misconception is that early terminations in particular are 'no big deal' because
the pregnancy is not very far advanced, and women are expected to
bounce back more quickly than they would after having their wisdom
teeth removed. The same psychological pain is involved in making the
decision as for terminations later in pregnancy, and there are the same
feelings of grief and loss.

Immediately after a termination, there may be a temporary feeling of
euphoria – the decision was made, the operation was carried out, and
you have survived the whole thing. After about 5–7 days, a deep depression can set in. This is partly because of hormonal confusion resulting
from the operation, rather like postnatal depression, and partly due to
the sheer emotional stress of the situation.

## MARKING THE EVENT

There are widely differing views amongst parents, health professionals,
and religious advisers about what is the right way to deal with a fetus
after it has been lost through medical termination, lethal abnormality,
miscarriage, or stillbirth. (This is not an issue in cases of surgical terminations, as there is no body to see or hold.) If the baby dies before
it reaches the gestation necessary for official birth registration, the need
for formal recognition and burial is not acknowledged in many places.
From the very beginning, the pregnancy has been real for the parents,
so it is confusing and upsetting to hear at the end that the baby did not
officially exist. Other people often adopt the positive approach and try

to get the parents to forget as quickly as possible and 'get on with life'. Yet forgetting is even harder when there is nothing to mark the event – no name, no grave, nothing. This is another reason why supportive counselling afterwards is so important. Even close friends and family may feel uncomfortable with the parents' need to grieve.

If the parents wish to do so, it is usually possible to have a special funeral service for the baby to mark its existence and to help parents begin the grieving process. Many hospital chaplains offer this service, regardless of the denomination of the parents; it can be an 'ecumenical' service. By the very nature of the offer of support, concern, and consideration for the parents' feelings it can be of great help. Some parents reject this idea initially because they want to 'get back to normal' as quickly as possible, but many eventually realize that such a service would help them in doing this.

## GRIEF

Termination for abnormality, miscarriage, stillbirth, neonatal death – these experiences are emotionally very traumatic at the time but also have lasting effects months or years later. People express and deal with feelings of grief in different ways. Your experience of grief may depend on several things – your relationship with your partner; the stage of pregnancy at which the event occurred; whether you have any other children or can have any more children; whether the pregnancy was wanted; your age and state of health; your experiences of grief in the past.

Everyone needs time to come to terms with what has happened, but the most important thing is being able to talk about how you feel with a supportive listener. You may have totally conflicting emotions such as depression and relief that make it difficult to talk to anyone. You may want desperately to talk to someone but find that other people avoid the subject because they feel uncomfortable, or they fear it will make you uncomfortable. Others who are unaware of or unsympathetic to your circumstances can ask painful questions. Feelings of guilt and shame may make you wary of talking to other people. This is why counselling and support groups are so valuable. Counsellors can help you to go over the medical facts and talk through your emotions without embarrassment, while support groups can provide the extremely reassuring feeling that you are not alone, and that there are people who understand what you are going through. Recovery time depends entirely on the individual. It is not unusual to feel sad and depressed years later. The expected delivery date is an especially difficult time that can bring back painful memories year after year.

Your self-image can suffer badly in these situations. You have lost a pregnancy, which can also lead to loss of confidence and feelings of failure and 'I can't do anything right'. Even formerly very confident people can feel uncertain and vulnerable afterwards and wonder, 'If this can happen, what else could go wrong for us?' If there were no obvious risk factors in your pregnancy but the outcome was the death of the baby, your whole view of the world can be turned upside down in a matter of weeks. Things seem to happen very quickly in the time leading up to the diagnosis or loss but, once the termination or funeral is over, time seems to stretch. It is not unusual to feel listless, lethargic, unable to concentrate on anything for a long time.

Plus, there is still a strong subconscious feeling in society that producing a baby confirms you are a 'real' man or woman. After a termination or loss the world around you suddenly seems filled with happy pregnant women and healthy little babies. You may find it unbearable to be around these people because they have achieved the feat of producing a healthy baby and they remind you of your 'failure'. There is no 'feat' or 'failure' involved at all. They embarked on the same biological process as you did; they just happened to be luckier. You are no less real than they are, and the recognition of this fact is an important step in recovery.

The desire to replace the pregnancy with a normal one can be very strong, but you may also be worried about your ability to cope if the same thing happened again. In general, people who have other children or who go on to have a healthy baby later cope better with the previous loss. However, it is not always easy to become pregnant again once you stop contraception. Women describe being obsessed with getting pregnant, while being afraid of the chance of having another abnormal pregnancy. You may become afraid of sex as the event which started all the problems, and feel that your partner 'got off lightly'.

You and your partner may find it difficult to communicate and understand each other's reactions. Men can show their grief in different ways or at different times to women. Many men prefer to deal with their feelings privately and are uncomfortable with a woman's open expressions of emotion. She feels that he is insensitive and uncaring – he feels impatient and victimized, the only target for her anger and frustration. Your relationship could change temporarily or permanently, but it appears that the most difficult time is between 3 and 6 months after the event.

Your anger may well be directed at the medical staff. It is not uncommon to feel that you have been let down by them, that they and their technology have failed you. Also, some parents do feel that they are not taken seriously, that their concerns are not given sufficient attention. In such situations, when you are drained by emotional stress, it can be very difficult to assert yourself. Regardless of how busy the medical staff is, it is perfectly reasonable to ask for as full an explanation as possible, and for your questions to be answered, even if the answer is, 'We don't know'.

## WHY US?

Even if both partners are in agreement about whether or not to continue with the pregnancy, there is often a search for a deeper explanation for the abnormality. Although this is a natural reaction, it can be fruitless and hurtful. For this reason, we want to reiterate a point made early on in this book: **most abnormalities occur randomly in people who cannot be associated with any risk factor whatsoever.** In almost all cases, the answer to the question, 'What could we have done to prevent this happening?' is 'Nothing'. It is not very comforting to think that you have so little control, but at least you can be reassured that neither action nor inaction on your part was in any way responsible for the outcome. That glass of wine, having sex late in the pregnancy, that spicy meal, not getting enough rest, getting too much rest, taking painkillers for a headache, going to a party where people were smoking – none of this will have had the least effect on your baby. You have been unlucky, just as someone who was struck by lightning is unlucky; there is no blame attached. It was a terrible accident, but there was absolutely no way to prevent it. You will speed the recovery process if you can support and comfort each other rather than pulling yourselves apart looking for a target for your sadness and disappointment.

## WHAT ABOUT THE FUTURE?

If you decide later that you might want to try again, there are some important considerations: the risk of recurrence, positive steps you can take; and methods of prenatal diagnosis. Genetic counsellors can discuss all of these issues with you.

If a single gene disorder has been diagnosed, the recurrence risk depends on whether it arose as a new mutation (dominant or some

X-linked), whether the parents are carriers, or whether there is a family history of the disease.

In the case of dominant conditions, if both parents are normal then there must have been a new mutation because only one affected copy of the gene is necessary to cause the disease. This means that the risk of recurrence is very low. Some X-linked conditions can arise as new mutations, which is the case if the mother is tested and found not to be a carrier. The recurrence risk in these cases is also very low.

If the parents are found to be carriers, or if there is a family history of the disease as described in Chapter 2, inherited single-gene disorders have a recurrence risk of either: 25 per cent (recessive); 50 per cent (dominant); 50 per cent of all male children (X-linked); or 100 per cent (rare cases such as those where both parents are affected by the same recessive condition).

For chromosome disorders, the recurrence risk depends on whether the abnormality was caused by a new mutation (97–98 per cent of cases) or whether the baby inherited an unbalanced rearrangement of the parents' chromosomes (2–3 per cent of cases). In the former case, the recurrence risk is very low, but the risk is higher in the latter case. This depends on the particular type of rearrangement, and your genetic counsellor can discuss your particular situation with you.

If a multifactorial condition has been diagnosed, the recurrence risk will usually be given as 2–5 per cent. These include such conditions as spina bifida, certain heart defects, and cases of cleft lip and palate that are not part of a specific syndrome. In cases of Down syndrome where the parents' chromosomes are normal, the recurrence risk is also 1 per cent. When dealing with a well known abnormality, your doctor can tell you these figures. For some lesser known conditions, expert genetic counselling may be needed, and this still may not provide you with a precise recurrence risk. Whatever risk factors are quoted may only apply to having another baby with the same partner. For example, if your baby had a recessive condition like cystic fibrosis and your next partner is not a carrier, then the recurrence risk drops from 25 to 0 per cent.

For some conditions, certain precautions should be taken before conception. If you have diabetes, you may need to change your insulin dose to obtain the best glucose control possible just before conception and during the first few weeks of pregnancy. Likewise, if you have had a fetus with spina bifida, you would be advised to take folate supplements in the same time period.

Some parents find that having a baby or fetus with an abnormality is so devastating that they choose not to have any more children, even to the point of sterilization. Alternatively, they may decide to adopt a child or undergo assisted conception using donor sperm or eggs to avoid the risk for certain hereditary conditions. Another option that may become increasingly important in the future is pre-implantation diagnosis. This involves *in vitro* fertilization with the parents' sperm and egg and removing some of the cells of the embryo at a very early stage for analysis. Only those embryos shown to be normal are put back into the mother's uterus.

Parents may really want to have more children but are so frightened of the possibility of recurrence that they put off the decision for a number of years. This can be good because new methods for prevention, diagnosis, and treatment may become available. However, this delay has its own problems because fertility declines, and the risks for some conditions increase, with the mother's age; there are also parental age limits on adoption and assisted conception programmes (as low as 35 years in some places).

The choice of prenatal testing methods in a later pregnancy may well be different from those used this time, depending on the type of abnormality detected. For example, if Down syndrome was diagnosed in the current pregnancy through amniocentesis in the second trimester, you might want an earlier diagnosis through CVS soon after 10 weeks next time. Similarly, if the fetus had anencephaly or spina bifida, you should have an ultrasound scan at 11–12 weeks in the next pregnancy.

If you think that you do want to try again, but are worried about the risks, your doctor or genetic counsellor should be able to explain these to you as well as any other options that exist. Knowledge of the previous condition can help a lot in planning a future pregnancy. One big advantage is that you will be able to think through all the risks and possible outcomes without being under pressure of time, consult specialists, and discuss your feelings at length with your partner. All of this can provide a strong emotional and mental foundation if the decision is made to try again.

## CONCLUSION

In the 3 years that it has taken us to write this book, a huge amount of progress has been made in the diagnosis and treatment of fetal abnormalities. This has led, of course, to a dramatic increase in the provision of testing services, which can only continue to increase in the next few years. Tests are being discovered and refined to become quicker and more accurate and the understanding of genetic disease is improving all the time. Communication with parents does not always improve with technology, however, and we hope that this book has been helpful to those in this situation.

# Glossary

Words in bold are defined in other entries in the glossary.

*AFP (alpha-fetoprotein).* This is the first protein produced by a developing baby. Its level in the mother's blood is measured to screen for possible **neural tube defects** and Down syndrome.

*AID (artificial insemination by donor).* This may be an option for couples at high risk of an inherited disease, such as when both partners are carriers. It involves inseminating the mother with sperm from a donor who is not a carrier.

*Amniocentesis.* A **diagnostic test** which involves taking a sample of the amniotic fluid for analysis.

*Base.* The base is the smallest unit of genetic material. Bases are joined together in pairs to make genes. Although small, the change of even a single base can cause disease.

*Chromosome.* The chromosome is the largest unit of genetic material. Every cell in the body has 46 of them. When eggs and sperm are formed, they each contain only 23 chromosomes, which combine at fertilization to make 46 and produce an embryo. Chromosomes can be damaged, or their numbers altered, when the egg and sperm are formed, which can result in abnormalities in the baby.

*Cordocentesis.* Another name for **fetal blood sampling**.

*CVS.* A **diagnostic test** that involves taking a sample of the placenta for analysis.

*Diagnostic test.* Diagnostic tests are performed to ascertain definitely whether or not a baby is affected by a certain condition. They are usually only offered to people who can be identified as at risk because of screening test results, family history of disease, or age of the mother.

*Disomy.* Another word for 'a pair'. The normal situation is to have a pair or disomy of each **chromosome**, one from the mother and one from the father.

*Dominant gene.* A dominant gene is the most assertive form of a gene, in contrast to 'recessive' genes. Only one copy of a dominant gene is needed for it to show itself or be 'expressed'.

*DNA (deoxyribonucleic acid).* The substance of which genes are made. Tests have been developed to analyse DNA for certain single gene disorders.

*Fetal blood sampling.* A **diagnostic test** that involves taking a sample of blood from the umbilical cord for analysis.

*Folic acid/folate.* A vitamin that is thought to be important in protecting against **neural tube defects** if taken just before conception and during early pregnancy.

*Gene.* The functional unit of DNA, made up of thousands of **bases**. Genes ultimately control every physical trait of the body. Some genes work alone, some work with other genes, and some are affected by factors in the environment.

*Genome.* The total genetic complement of an organism. The human genome comprises 33 000 000 000 **bases**.

*Gestational age.* The number of weeks that the baby has been 'gestating' or developing, usually calculated from the date of the mother's last period.

*Haemoglobin.* The molecule that transports oxygen in the bloodstream. Thalassaemia and sickle cell disease are single gene disorders that affect the structure of haemoglobin and result in severe anaemia.

*Invasive test.* Invasive tests involve taking a sample of fluid or tissue from within the womb – the placenta, the amniotic fluid, blood from the umbilical cord, etc. With the exception of ultrasound, all diagnostic tests are invasive and therefore carry a risk of miscarriage.

In vitro *fertilization.* This involves combining the egg and sperm outside the mother's body and then implanting the embryo in the uterus. It forms part of the **pre-implantation diagnosis** procedure.

*Karyotype.* A picture of an individual's **chromosomes**. It is produced from a sample of cells from the baby or parents to check for abnormalities in the number of chromosomes or their appearance (pieces missing or rearranged).

*Multifactorial conditions.* These are diseases that result from the interaction of **genes** and environmental factors. There may be several genes and several factors involved which can be very difficult to unravel. Certain instances of cleft lip and palate and heart defects are thought to be multifactorial.

*Mutation.* This literally means 'change'. In a genetic context it means a change affecting a **gene**. Only one or several **bases** may be affected. Some mutations have no noticeable effect, some are beneficial, and some cause disease.

*Negative test result.* This means that the condition the test was designed to detect has *not* been found.

*Neural tube defects.* These result when the nervous system does not develop properly. Blood vessels are left exposed, which leads to a higher than normal amount of **AFP** leaking out. This is why the level of **AFP** is measured to screen for possible neural tube defects. Anencephaly and spina bifida are examples of neural tube defects.

*Positive test result.* This means that the condition the test was designed to detect *has* been found.

*Pre-implantation diagnosis.* Another option for couples at high risk for passing on an inherited disease to their baby. *In vitro* **fertilization** is carried out, the embryos are tested for the condition, and only unaffected embryos are implanted in the uterus.

*Recessive gene.* The least assertive form of a gene, contrasted with **dominant genes**. Recessive genes can be invisible or they can affect the expression of the dominant gene. Usually the baby must inherit two recessive disease genes, one from each parent, to be affected by the condition.

*Screening test.* Screening tests are performed routinely for everyone attending an antenatal clinic, although not all of the tests described in this book will be offered everywhere. Screening tests are designed to identify mothers with a higher than average risk of having a baby affected by an abnormality. They include taking a medical history, testing the mother's blood, and doing ultrasound scans.

*Serum screening for Down syndrome (also known as the triple test).* A low level of **AFP** in the mother's blood and certain levels of two other hormones are associated with an increased risk of Down syndrome. This test measures the levels of these substances. Because it is a screening test, the result is an expression of risk rather than a diagnosis.

*Sex-linked gene.* See **X-linked gene**.

*Teratogen.* Substances that can affect adversely the baby's development in the womb. Infections, X-rays, and drugs are examples of teratogens.

*Triple test.* See **Serum screening for Down syndrome.**

*Triploidy.* Sometimes instead of there being a **disomy** or pair of each **chromosome**, the baby receives three copies of *every* chromosome. This condition is known as triploidy and is lethal.

*Trisomy.* Instead of having a pair or **disomy** of each chromosome, the baby receives three copies of *one* chromosome. For example, Trisomy 21 (Down syndrome) means that the baby has three copies of chromosome number 21.

*Ultrasound.* This is a testing method that is used both for **screening** and **diagnosis.** It works by using sound waves interpreted by a computer to build up an image of the baby. It is not **invasive** and therefore does not pose a risk to the baby, but its usefulness varies with the skill of the operator and the equipment available.

*X-linked gene.* Genes found on the X **chromosome.** Females have two X chromosomes and males have an X and a Y. Some disease genes such as those for haemophilia and Duchenne muscular dystrophy are located on the X chromosome.

# Appendix 1

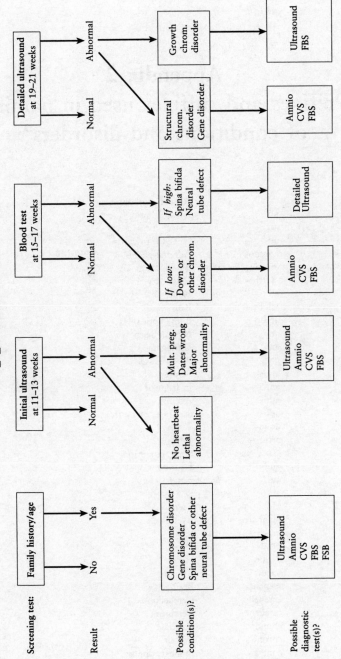

| Screening test: | Family history/age | Initial ultrasound at 11–13 weeks | Blood test at 15–17 weeks | Detailed ultrasound at 19–21 weeks |
|---|---|---|---|---|
| **Result** | No / Yes | Normal / Abnormal | Normal / Abnormal | Normal / Abnormal |
| **Possible condition(s)?** | Chromosome disorder Gene disorder Spina bifida or other neural tube defect | No heartbeat Lethal abnormality / Mult. preg. Dates wrong Major abnormality | *If low:* Down or other chrom. disorder / *If high:* Spina bifida Neural tube defect | Structural chrom. disorder Gene disorder / Growth chrom. disorder |
| **Possible diagnostic test(s)?** | Ultrasound Amnio CVS FBS FSB | Ultrasound Amnio CVS FBS | Amnio CVS FBS / Detailed Ultrasound | Amnio CVS FBS / Ultrasound FBS |

# Appendix 2
# Prefixes and suffixes used in naming of conditions and disorders*

| | |
|---|---|
| a- | Absent, without |
| ab- | Away from |
| acro- | Extremity |
| ad- | Next to, towards |
| adreno- | Adrenal glands |
| -aemia, -emia | Blood |
| -aesthesia | Sensitivity |
| albi - | White |
| -algia | Pain |
| ambi- | Both, both sides |
| an- | Not, deficient |
| ana- | Up, again |
| angio- | Blood vessels |
| ante- | Before |
| antero- | In front of |
| anti- | Against |
| apo- | Separate, away from |
| aqua- | Water |
| arthro- | Joints |
| -asis, -asia | State, condition |
| audio- | Hearing |
| auri- | Ear |
| auto- | Self |
| bi- | Two |
| blepharo- | Eyelids |
| brachy- | Short |
| brady- | Slow |
| cardio- | Heart |
| -cele | Tumour |
| -cephal | Brain, head. |
| cerebello- | Cerebellum |
| cerebro- | Cerebrum |
| chondro- | Cartilage |
| chrom- | Colour |
| contra- | Against, opposite |

| | |
|---|---|
| cortico- | Outer layer |
| costo- | Ribs |
| cranio- | Cranium |
| cyclo- | Circular |
| cyto- | Cells |
| -dactyl- | Fingers, toes |
| di- | Twice, double |
| dia- | Through, across |
| diplo- | Twofold |
| dis- | Separate, apart |
| dys- | Impaired, difficult, painful |
| ecto- | Outer or outside |
| -ectomy | Cutting out |
| encephalo- | Brain |
| endo- | Internal, within |
| epi- | Upon, above |
| ex- | Out |
| exo- | Situated outside |
| extra- | In addition to |
| facio- | Face |
| fibro- | Fibrous |
| gastro- | Stomach |
| genito- | Genital organs |
| glosso- | Tongue |
| glyco- | Sugar |
| gnath- | Jaw |
| haem- | Blood |
| hemi- | Half |
| hepato- | Liver |
| hetero- | Different |
| holo- | Whole, complete |
| homeo-, homo- | Same or similar |
| hydro- | Water |
| hyper- | More than normal, excessive |
| hypo- | Less than normal, lacking |
| -ia, -iasis | Condition of |
| infra- | Below or under |
| inter- | Between, among |
| intra- | Inside, within |
| intro- | Into, inward |
| iso- | Equal |
| kine- | Movement |
| laryngo- | Larynx |
| lento- | Lens of the eye |
| leuco- | White |
| macro- | Large |
| mal- | Bad, faulty |
| mega-, megalo- | Great |
| -melia | Limb |

| meso-          | Middle                          |
|----------------|---------------------------------|
| meta-          | Beyond, change                  |
| micro-         | Small                           |
| mono-          | Single                          |
| muco-          | Mucous                          |
| multi-         | Many                            |
| my-, myo-      | Muscle                          |
| narco-         | Sleep                           |
| neo-           | New                             |
| nephro-        | Kidneys                         |
| neuro-         | Nerves                          |
| noct-          | Night                           |
| oculo-         | Eye                             |
| -oid           | Resembling                      |
| oligo-         | Few, slight                     |
| -oma           | Tumour                          |
| omni-          | All                             |
| -opia          | Vision                          |
| ophth-         | Eye                             |
| ortho-         | Straight, upright               |
| -ose, -ous     | Abounding in, characterized by  |
| -osis          | Condition, especially disease   |
| osteo-         | Bone                            |
| oto-           | Ear                             |
| pachy-         | Thick                           |
| palato-        | Palate                          |
| pan-           | All                             |
| para-          | Beyond, beside                  |
| patho-, -pathy | Disease, disorder               |
| peri-          | Around                          |
| phon-          | Sound                           |
| photo-         | Light                           |
| physio-        | Natural                         |
| -plasia        | Construction, development       |
| -plegia        | Paralysis                       |
| poly-          | Many                            |
| post-          | After, behind                   |
| pre-           | Before, in time or order        |
| pro-           | In front of, before in time     |
| proto-         | Original or first               |
| pseudo-        | False                           |
| psycho-        | The mind                        |
| pykno-, pycno- | Dense, close together           |
| pyro-          | Heat                            |
| quadri-        | Four                            |
| re-            | Back again, repeated            |
| retro-         | Backwards, behind               |
| rhino-         | Nose                            |
| rhizo-         | Root-like                       |

| | |
|---|---|
| scler- | Hard |
| semi- | Half |
| spleno- | Spleen |
| sub- | Under, below |
| super- | On the top, more |
| supra- | Above or upper |
| sym- | Associated with, together |
| syn- | Together |
| tachy- | Rapid |
| -taxia, taxic | Co-ordination, movement |
| tele- | Distance |
| tetra- | Group of four |
| thermo- | Heat, temperature |
| -tomy | Cutting |
| toxo- | Poison |
| trans- | Through, across |
| trich- | Hair |
| -trophy | Nutrition, growth |
| ultra- | Extreme, excess |
| uni- | One |
| -uria | Urine |
| xan- | Yellow |
| xero- | Dry |

* Reproduced with permission from the Birth Defects Foundation

# Appendix 3
# Groups offering help and support

This is just a small selection of the groups which exist. More can be found through your local doctor, hospital, counsellor, or telephone directory.

**Britain**

Alcohol Concern
275 Grays Inn Rd, London WC1 8QF

Birth Defects Foundation
Chelsea House, Westgate, London W5 1DR

Cystic Fibrosis Trust
Alexandra House, 5 Blythe Rd, Bromley, Kent BR1 3RS

Down Syndrome Association
155 Mitcham Rd, London SW17 9PG

Association for Spina Bifida and Hydrocephalus
ASBAH House, 42 Park Rd, Peterborough PE1 2UQ

Haemophilia Society
123 Westminster Bridge Rd, London SE1 7HR

Muscular Dystrophy Society of Great Britain and Northern Ireland
7–11 Prescott Place, London SW4 6BS

National Childbirth Trust
Alexandra House, Oldham Terrace, Acton, London W3 6NH

Neurofibromatosis Society
120 London Rd, Kingston-upon-Thames, Surrey KT2 6QJ

Retinitis Pigmentosa Society
Pond House, Lillingstone, Dayrell, Bucks MK18 5AS

Royal Society for Mentally Handicapped Children and Adults
(MENCAP)
National Centre, 123 Golden Lane, London EC1Y 0RT

Stillbirth and Neonatal Death Society (SANDS)
28 Portland Place, London W1N 4DE

Support After Termination for Fetal Abnormality (SATFA)
29–30 Soho Sq, London W1V 6JB

The Spastics Society
12 Park Crescent, London W1N 4EQ


**North America**

American Cleft Palate Education Foundation
331, Salk Hall, University of Pittsburgh, Pittsburgh, PA 15261

Alliance of Genetic Support Groups
35, Wisconsin Circl, Suite 440, Chevy Chase, MD 20815

Association for Children with Down Syndrome
2616 Martin Avenue, Bellmore, NY 11710-3196

Charcot–Marie–Tooth Association
Crozer Mills Enterprise Centre, 600 Upland Avenue, Upland,
PA 19015

The Chromosome 18 Registry and Research Society
6302 Fox Head, San Antonio, TX 78247

Cornelia de Lange Syndrome Foundation Inc.
60 Dyer Avenue, Collinsville, CT 06022-1273

Crouzon's/Meniere's Support Network
2375 East Valentine #9, Prescott, AZ 86303-3122

Cystinosis Foundation Inc.
17, Lake Avenue, Piedmont, CA 94611

FACES, The National Association for Craniofacially Handicapped
P.O. Box 11082, Chattanooga, TN 37401

Klinefelter Syndrome KS and Associates
P.O. Box 119, Roseville, CA 95661-0119

March of Dimes Birth Defects Foundation
National Office, 1275, Manwaronek Avenue, White Plains,
NY 10605
(Produces many publications including books, leaflets, special topics
packages, audiocassettes and films)

Mucopolysaccharidoses and Mucolipidoses National MPS Society Inc.
17, Kraemer Street, Hicksville, NY 11801

MUMS Mothers United for Moral Support Inc. (a support group for
the families of a child with any disability)
15, Custer Court, Green Bay, WI 54310

National Association of Albinism and Hypopigmentation
1500 Locust Street, Suite 1816, Philadelphia, PA 19102

National Institute of Neurological and Communicative Disorders
and Stroke
Building 31, Room 8A-06, National Institutes of Health, Bethesda,
MD 20892

The National Neurofibromatosis Society
National Office, 141, Fifth Avenue, Suite 7-S, New York,
NY 10010-7105

National Tay–Sachs and Allied Diseases Association
385, Elliott Street, Newton, MA 02164

National Tuberous Sclerosis Association Inc.
4351, Garden City Drive, Suite 660, Landover, MD 20785

Prader-Willi Syndrome Association National Office
6490 Excelsior Boulevard, E102, St Lois Park, MN 55426

Tourette Syndrome Association
42–40 Bell Boulevard, Bayride, NY 11361

Sotos Syndrome Support Association (SSSA)
797, W. Lockwood Boulevard, St Louis, MO 63122

Spina Bifida Association of America
1700 Rockville Pike, Suite 540, Rockville, MD 20852

# Appendix 4
# Bibliography

Borgaonker, D.S. (1991). *Chromosomal variation in man: a catalogue of chromosomal variants and anomalies*, (6th edn). Wiley-Liss, London.

Brock, D.J.H., Rodeck, C.H., and Ferguson-Smith, M.A. (eds) (1992). *Prenatal diagnosis and screening*. Churchill-Livingstone, Edinburgh.

Chard, T. and Richards, M.P.M. (1992). *Obstetrics in the 1990s: current controversies*. MacKeith Press, London.

Drife, J.O. and Donnai, D. (1991). *Antenatal diagnosis of fetal abnormalities*. Springer-Verlag, Heidelberg.

Gabbe, S.G., Niebyl, J.R., and Simpson, J.L. (1991). *Obstetrics: normal and problem pregnancies*. Churchill Livingstone, New York.

Jones, K.L. (1988). *Smith's recognisable patterns of human malformations*, (4th edn). Saunders, London.

Lilford, R.J. (1989). *Prenatal diagnosis and prognosis*. Butterworth, Guildford.

Moore, K.L. (1988). *The developing human: clinically oriented embryology*, (4th edn). Saunders, London.

Neilson, J.P. and Chambers, S.E. (1993). *Obstetric ultrasound I*. Oxford University Press, Oxford.

Simpson, J.L., Golbus, M.S., Martin, A.O., and Sarto, G.E. (1982). *Genetics in obstetrics and gynaecology*. Grune and Stratton, London.

# Further Reading

Ardetti, R., Duelli, R., Duelli Klein, R., and Minden, S. (1985). *Test tube women. What future motherhood?* Pandora, London.

Burke, L., Himmelweit, S., and Vines, G. (1990). *Tomorrow's child: reproductive technologies in the 90s.* Virago, London.

de Crespigny, L. and Dredge, R. (1991). *Which tests for my unborn baby?* Oxford University Press, Melbourne.

Goodman, R.M. (1986). *Planning for a healthy baby.* Oxford University Press, New York.

Harris, A. (1991). *Cystic fibrosis: the facts.* Oxford University Press, Oxford.

Holmes, H.B., Hoskins, B.B., and Gross, M. (1981). *The custom-made child: women centered perspectives.* Humana Press, New York.

Kevles, D.J. (1985). *In the name of eugenics: genetics and the uses of human heredity.* Penguin, London.

Raphael-Leff, J. (1991). *Psychological processes of childbearing.* Chapman and Hall, London.

*Support after termination for fetal abnormality: a parent's handbook.* Available from SATFA (see list of support groups – Britain).

Selikowitz, M. (1990). *Down syndrome: the facts.* Oxford University Press, Oxford.

# Index

Index